O D

OXFORD DIABETES LIBR

Type 2 Diabetes

Jet

Joint Education and Training Library

This book is to be returned on or before the last date stamped below. Overdue charges will be incurred by the late return of books.

Renew in person, by phone (01270 612538, or internal x2538/3172) or online at: http://libcat.chester.ac.uk (NHS staff ask for password)

Oxford University Press makes no representation, express or implied, that the drug dosages in this book are correct. Readers must therefore always check the product information and clinical procedures with the most up-to-date published product information and data sheets provided by the manufacturers and the most recent codes of conduct and safety regulations. The authors and the publishers do not accept responsibility or legal liability for any errors in the text or for the misuse or misapplication of material in this work.

▶ Except where otherwise stated, drug doses and recommendations are for the non-pregnant adult who is not breast-feeding.

O D L

OXFORD DIABETES LIBRARY

Type 2 Diabetes

SECOND EDITION

Edited by

Professor Anthony H. Barnett

University of Birmingham, and
Heart of England NHS
Foundation Trust,
Birmingham, UK

OXFORD
UNIVERSITY PRESS

JET LIBRARY

OXFORD
UNIVERSITY PRESS

Great Clarendon Street, Oxford OX2 6DP,
United Kingdom

Oxford University Press is a department of the University of Oxford.
It furthers the University's objective of excellence in research, scholarship,
and education by publishing worldwide. Oxford is a registered trade mark of
Oxford University Press in the UK and in certain other countries

First Edition published 2008
Second Edition published 2012

Impression: 1

British Library Cataloguing in Publication Data

Data available

Library of Congress Cataloging in Publication Data

Data available

ISBN 978–0–19–959617–1

Printed in Great Britain by
Ashford Colour Press Ltd., Gosport, Hampshire

Contents

Preface to the first edition

When the author was a medical student textbooks told us that there were around 30 million people worldwide with diabetes. These numbers have now swelled to around 250 million and will reach 370 million within the next 20 years. This massive increase is mainly accounted for by an increase in numbers of patients with type 2 diabetes who now represent around 95% of new cases. The major driver for type 2 diabetes is the increasing prevalence of overweight and obesity, both in the developed and developing World. Diabetes is also associated with a whole range of major long term complications, the most important of which is a significantly increased risk of cardiovascular events (particularly myocardial infarction). In the UK and elsewhere, diabetes is also the commonest cause of blindness in the working population, the single commonest reason for chronic renal failure and need for dialysis and the single commonest reason for non-traumatic lower limb amputation. The costs of diabetes are high and rising.

In recent years, we have come to understand much more about the pathogenesis of type 2 diabetes. This includes the realisation that both insulin resistance and pancreatic islet cell dysfunction are vital components in development of type 2 diabetes in the vast majority of patients. In addition, deteriorating pancreatic beta cell function is responsible for the progressive nature of type 2 diabetes.

We also now have a large and impressive evidence base to help us manage this condition, particularly from the point of view of cardio-vascular risk factor intervention and indeed one needs now to be asking the question "Why is this patient with type 2 diabetes not on a statin, antihypertensives and low dose aspirin (once blood pressure is controlled)" rather than "Should this patient be on. . .". Indeed, with appropriate interventions it is possible to reach recommended targets for cholesterol and blood pressure in the majority of patients. Achieving tight glycaemic control is commonly much more challenging and indeed mean HbA_{1c} across the World tends to be uniformly bad! There are a whole range of reasons for this and importantly this includes the fact that type 2 diabetes is a progressive disease and that none of the traditional agents used in management have been shown to slow or reverse that progression.

In this small book aimed at the multiprofessional primary care team, I have attempted to focus on glycaemia management, although importantly there are chapters on multiple cardiovascular risk factor intervention to ensure that the book is balanced. In recent years there has, however, been much interest in new therapies for diabetes *per se* and indeed we have moved far from the era when only met-formin, sulfonylurea and insulin were available as pharmacotherapies for type 2 diabetes. Several new treatments have appeared on the market including the thiazolidinediones (glitazones), and the very recently introduced incretin mimetics and DPP-4 inhibitors with a promise of many other interesting compounds to come in the future. There have also been important advances in insulin therapy per se and also in mode of insulin delivery.

It has been my great pleasure to invite a range of experts from the diabetes world in the UK to contribute chapters to this small book. I have not tried to comprehensively cover the whole field of type 2 diabetes but there are chapters covering complications and costs of the condition; lifestyle intervention as an important part of man-age-ment; multiple cardiovascular risk factor intervention; managing glycaemia using current oral agents; review of management of type 2 diabetes with insulin; managing glycaemia with recently introduced and future therapies. The final chapter looks at the challenges to good diabetes care, including the role of the multiprofessional team and different educational approaches.

Each chapter has been written by a recognised expert in the field and most are concerned with day-to-day management of diabetes patients. This means that the authorship has included a GP, a Diabetes. Nurse Consultant, a person with an interest in behavioural therapy, a Diabetes Specialist Nurse and Consultant Diabetologists. Given that the book is multi-author there will inevitably be some overlap between the chapters, although I have tried to keep this to a minimum. I believe that the result is a highly readable and extremely practical educational tool to help colleagues in primary care who are part of the multiprofessional team looking after patients with diabetes.

Anthony Barnett,
January 2008

Symbols and abbreviations

ACCORD	Action to Control Cardiovascular Risk in Diabetes
ACE	angiotensin-converting enzyme
ADA	American Diabetes Association
ADOPT	A Diabetes Outcome Progression Trial
ADVANCE	Action in Diabetes and Vascular disease: preterAx and diamicroN-MR Controlled Evaluation
AER	albumin excretion rate
AHA	American Heart Association
ATP	adenosine triphosphate
BMI	body mass index
CIT	conventional insulin treatment
CTT	Cholesterol Treatment Trialists
CVD	cardiovascular disease
DARTS	Diabetes Audit and Research in Tayside Scotland
DAWN	Diabetes Attitudes Wishes and Needs
DCCT	Diabetes Control and Complications Trial
DESMOND	Diabetes Education and Self-Management for Ongoing and Newly Diagnosed
DPPIV	Dipeptidyl peptidase-4
DREAM	Diabetes Reduction Assessment with ramipril and rosiglitazone Medication
EASD	European Association for the Study of Diabetes
ECG	electrocardiography
eGFR	estimated glomerular filtration rate
FDA	Federal Drug Administration
GIP	gastric inhibitory polypeptide
GFR	glomerular filtration rate
GI	gastro-intestinal
GI	glycaemic index
GIP	glucose-dependent insulinotropic polypeptide
GL	glucose-lowering

GLP	glucagon-like peptide-1
HDL	high density lipoproteins
HOT	Hypertension Optimal Treatment
IDF	International Diabetes Federation
IFG	impaired fasting glycaemia
IGT	impaired glucose tolerance
ISICA	International Study of Insulin and Cancer
JUPITER	Justification for the Use of statins in Prevention: an Intervention Trial Evaluating Rosuvastatin
LCD	low calorie diets
LDL	low density lipoproteins
LDL-C	low-density lipoprotein cholesterol
LEAD	Liraglutide Effect and Action in Diabetes
LFD	low fat diets
MIT	multiple insulin injection treatment
NEFA	non-esterified fatty acid levels
NICE	National Institute for Health and Clinical Excellence
NPH	neutral protamine Hagedorn (isophane insulin)
NSF	National Service Framework
ODA	oral diabetes agent
OHA	oral hypoglycaemic agents
PPAR	peroxisome proliferator-activated receptors
PROactive	PROspective pioglitAzone Clinical Trial In macroVascular Events
RECORD	Rosiglitazone Evaluated for Cardiac Outcomes and Regulation of Glycaemia in Diabetes
SNS	sympathetic nervous system stimulation
STOP-NIDDM	Study to Prevent Non-Insulin Dependent Diabetes Mellitus
TZD	thiazolidinediones
UGDP	University Group Diabetes Program
UKPDS	UK Prospective Diabetes Study
VADT	Veteran Administration Diabetes Trial
VLCD	very low calorie diets
VLDL	very low density lipoproteins

Contributors

Professor Clifford J Bailey
Professor of Clinical Science,
Diabetes Research Group,
School of Life and Health
Sciences, Aston University,
Birmingham, UK

Professor Anthony Barnett
University of Birmingham, and
Heart of England NHS
Foundation Trust,
Birmingham, UK

Dr Cristina Bianchi
Clinical Researcher,
University of Pisa, Department
of Endocrinology &
Metabolism—Section of
Metabolic Diseases and
Diabetes, Pisa, Italy

Dr Richard A Chudleigh
University of Wales College of
Medicine, Diabetes Research
Unit, Academic Centre,
Llandough Hospital,
Penarth, UK

Dr Caroline Day
Diabetes Research Group,
School of Life and Health
Sciences, Aston University,
Birmingham, UK

Professor Miles Fisher
Consultant Physician, Diabetes
Centre, Glasgow Royal
Infirmary, Glasgow, UK

Dr Roger Gadsby
GP and Associate Clinical
Professor, Warwick Medical
School, University of Warwick,
Coventry, UK

Jill Hill
Diabetes Nurse Consultant,
Community Diabetes Team,
Eastern Birmingham PCT,
PAK Medical Centre,
Birmingham, UK

Dr Katarina Kos
Clinical Lecturer,
Diabetes and Endocrinology
Clinical Research Group,
University Hospital Aintree,
Liverpool, UK

Dr Cathy E Lloyd
Senior Lecturer, Faculty of
Health and Social Care,
The Open University,
Milton Keynes, UK

Professor David R Owens
Consultant Diabetologist,
University of Wales College of
Medicine, Diabetes Research
Unit, Academic Centre,
Llandough Hospital, Penarth, UK

Dr Rajesh Peter
University of Wales College of
Medicine, Diabetes Research
Unit, Academic Centre,
Llandough Hospital,
Penarth, UK,

Professor Stefano Del Prato

University of Pisa, Department of Endocrinology & Metabolism—Section of Metabolic Diseases and Diabetes, Pisa, Italy

Dr Santosh Shankarnarayan

Research Fellow, Royal Liverpool University Hospital, Liverpool, UK

Dr Gayatri Sreemantula

Specialist Registrar, Royal Liverpool University Hospital, Liverpool, UK

Dr Sarah Steven

Clinical Research Fellow, Magnetic Resonance Centre, Campus for Ageing and Health, University of Newcastle, Newcastle upon Tyne, UK

Dr Abd A Tahrani

Clinical Research Fellow, School of Clinical and Experimental Medicine, College of Medical and Dental Sciences, University of Birmingham, Birmingham, UK

Dr Roy Taylor

Professor of Medicine and Metabolism, Director, Magnetic Resonance Centre, Campus for Ageing and Health, University of Newcastle, Newcastle upon Tyne, UK

Professor Jiten P Vora

Consultant Physician, Endocrinologist, Royal Liverpool University Hospital, Liverpool, UK

Jackie Webb

Diabetes Specialist Nurse Manager, Department of Diabetes and Endocrinology, Birmingham Heartlands Hospital, Birmingham, UK

Professor John PH Wilding

Professor of Medicine, Diabetes and Endocrinology Clinical Research Group, University Hospital Aintree, Liverpool, UK

Chapter 1

Complications and costs of diabetes

Anthony Barnett

Key points

- Cardiovascular disease kills around 80% of all type 2 diabetic patients, many prematurely
- Diabetes is the commonest cause of:
  - blindness in the working population of the UK
  - chronic renal failure and need for dialysis
  - non-traumatic lower limb amputation
- Eighty percent of the costs of diabetes relate to the long-term complications
- There is a large and impressive evidence base for vascular risk reduction in diabetes patients.

1.1 Introduction

As a public health issue, diabetes presents two major problems—the sheer weight of numbers of patients and the long-term complications of the condition which can be devastating, leading to premature mortality and greatly increased risk of cardiovascular disease, blindness, kidney failure and amputation. In this chapter, I will consider the epidemiology, aetiology and consequences of both micro- and macrovascular disease as well as the costs of treatment.

1.2 Cardiovascular disease and type 2 diabetes

The co-occurrence of several cardiovascular risk factors including hypertension, dyslipidaemia and glucose intolerance in the same person has been noted for many years. Gerry Reaven put this relationship on a firm scientific footing in 1988 when he propounded his 'syndrome X' hypothesis (Reaven, 1988). He suggested that this co-occurrence of risk factors was due to a primary underlying abnormality, 'insulin resistance' (resistance of the body to the biological actions of insulin) (Figure 1.1). He proposed that insulin resistance led to the development of hyperinsulinaemia with an associated dylipidaemic profile with increases in low and very low density lipoproteins (LDL and VLDL) and a reduction in the anti-atherogenic fraction high density lipoproteins (HDL). These changes are recognized as a rise in plasma triglycerides and low HDL levels—highly atherogenic and commonly associated with type 2 diabetes.

Hyperinsulinaemia is also associated with hypertension, perhaps through increased sodium reabsorption from the proximal renal tubules and increased sympathetic nervous system stimulation (SNS). Reaven also proposed that in many individuals the pancreas would eventually be unable to secrete enough insulin to overcome the insulin resistance, contributing to pancreatic B-cell dysfunction, insulin deficiency and the development of impaired glucose tolerance and type 2 diabetes.

This syndrome of 'chronic cardiovascular risk/syndrome X' has since become known as the 'metabolic syndrome' and its development strongly correlates with central or visceral adiposity (i.e. increased fat within the abdomen, around the organs and within the liver, heart and skeletal muscles). This is measured clinically as an increase in waist circumference (Despres et al., 2001). Several organizations and professional bodies have tried to more precisely define metabolic syndrome (WHO, 1999; National Cholesterol Education Program, 2002; IDF, 2005). All definitions require at least three values to be outside the recommended ranges from the following: expanded waist circumference and/or increased body mass

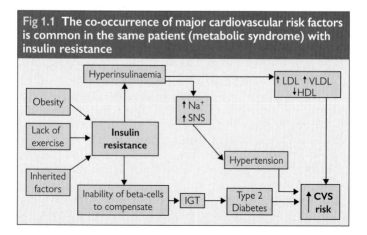

Fig 1.1 **The co-occurrence of major cardiovascular risk factors is common in the same patient (metabolic syndrome) with insulin resistance**

Fig 1.2 The IDF definition of metabolic syndrome requires expanded waist circumference as a necessary factor for diagnosis. Reproduced with permission from the International Diabetes Federation, www.idf.org

- Abdominal obesity (Europids: ♂ WC >94 cm, ♀ WC >80 cm), plus any two of the following (or treatment for):

– Elevated TG:	≥ 1.7 mmol/l
– Reduced HDL-cholesterol:	< 1.03 mmol/l (♂)
	< 1.29 mmol/l (♀)
– Raised BP:	≥ 130/85 mmHg
– Raised fasting plasma glucose:	≥ 5.6 mmol/l

index (BMI), low HDL cholesterol, raised triglycerides, raised blood pressure and glucose intolerance. More recently, the International Diabetes Federation (IDF) has recommended that an expanded waist circumference is a pre-requisite for the diagnosis of metabolic syndrome and that the reference ranges should be adjusted depending on ethnicity, with lower values in populations such as South Asian, Japanese and Chinese groups (IDF, 2005) (Figure 1.2).

1.3 Waist circumference, central obesity and cardiovascular/diabetes risk

Central obesity is just as profound a marker of cardiovascular risk as the other classical cardiovascular risk factors (Yusuf et al., 2004) (Figure 1.3). Waist circumference is our best clinical correlate for central/visceral adiposity. Fat cells (particularly those found centrally) are metabolically active and, in excess, are associated with increased release of free fatty acids, which are more resistant to the metabolic effects of insulin and more sensitive to lipolytic hormones (Jensen et al., 1989). An increased delivery of free fatty acids to the liver is associated with reduced insulin binding to liver cells and impaired insulin action leading to increased hepatic glucose production. There is also decreased utilization of free fatty acids in skeletal muscle. Fat cells also produce adipocytokines, including adiponectin, resistin, tumour necrosis factor α (TNF-α) and plasminogen activator inhibitor 1 (PAI-1) (McTernan & Kumar, 2004). Normally, there is a careful balance between various adipocytokines. Low concentrations of adiponectin are consistently found in populations at high cardiovascular risk and are associated with insulin resistance and hyperinsulinaemia.

There is also preliminary evidence that increased expression of resistin from visceral fat is associated with insulin resistance, and

Fig 1.3 Central obesity is a major independent risk factor for myocardial infarction (reproduced with permission from Yusuf et al., 2004)

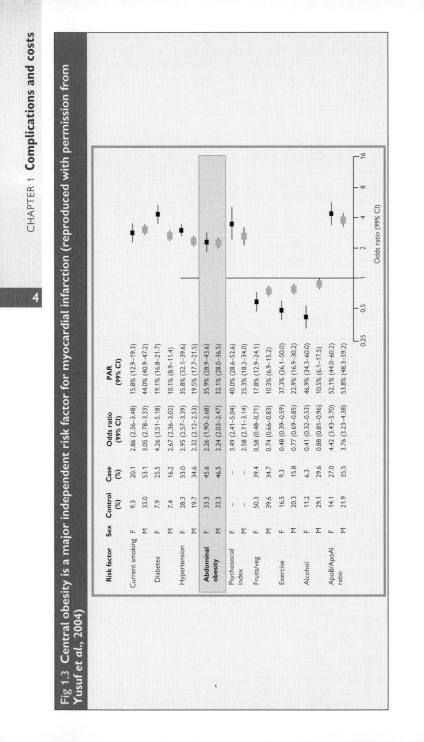

Risk factor	Sex	Control (%)	Case (%)	Odds ratio (99% CI)	PAR (99% CI)
Current smoking	F	9.3	20.1	2.86 (2.36–3.48)	15.8% (12.9–19.3)
	M	33.0	53.1	3.05 (2.78–3.33)	44.0% (40.9–47.2)
Diabetes	F	7.9	25.5	4.26 (3.51–5.18)	19.1% (16.8–21.7)
	M	7.4	16.2	2.67 (2.36–3.02)	10.1% (8.9–11.4)
Hypertension	F	28.3	53.0	2.95 (2.57–3.39)	35.8% (32.1–39.6)
	M	19.7	34.6	2.32 (2.12–2.53)	19.5% (17.7–21.5)
Abdominal obesity	F	33.3	45.6	2.26 (1.90–2.68)	35.9% (28.9–43.6)
	M	33.3	46.5	2.24 (2.03–2.47)	32.1% (28.0–36.5)
Psychosocial index	F	–	–	3.49 (2.41–5.04)	40.0% (28.6–52.6)
	M	–	–	2.58 (2.11–3.14)	25.3% (18.2–34.0)
Fruits/veg	F	50.3	39.4	0.58 (0.48–0.71)	17.8% (12.9–24.1)
	M	39.6	34.7	0.74 (0.66–0.83)	10.3% (6.9–15.2)
Exercise	F	16.5	9.3	0.48 (0.39–0.59)	37.3% (26.1–50.0)
	M	20.3	15.8	0.77 (0.69–0.85)	22.9% (16.9–30.2)
Alcohol	F	11.2	6.3	0.41 (0.32–0.53)	46.9% (34.3–60.0)
	M	29.1	29.6	0.88 (0.81–0.96)	10.5% (6.1–17.5)
ApoB/ApoAl ratio	F	14.1	27.0	4.42 (3.43–5.70)	52.1% (44.0–60.2)
	M	21.9	35.5	3.76 (3.23–4.38)	53.8% (48.3–59.2)

Odds ratio (99% CI)

other inflammatory cytokines such as TNF-α have also been implicated (McTernan & Kumar, 2004). Excess visceral fat appears, therefore, to be associated with the development of insulin resistance and atherogenic dyslipidaemia and increased atheroma formation and type 2 diabetes, through the dual mechanism of increased free fatty acid production and adipocytokine imbalance.

1.4 Implications for type 2 diabetes and cardiovascular disease

Whilst diabetes *per se* is not essential for the diagnosis of metabolic syndrome, most patients with type 2 diabetes have metabolic syndrome and even those who do not have diabetes are at significantly increased risk of developing it. The prevalence of metabolic syndrome increases with age and also shows large ethnic variations. In the USA there is a 22% prevalence of metabolic syndrome in the general population, but it is much higher in African American women and Hispanics (Ford *et al.*, 2002). Other studies have shown similarly high levels in South Asian populations, particularly on migration to Western countries (Barnett *et al.*, 2006). These findings are consistent with the much higher risk of diabetes and to an extent cardiovascular disease (particularly in South Asians) seen in these populations.

Diabetes *per se* is a major and independent risk factor for cardiovascular disease (Barnett & O'Gara, 2004). Others, including hypertension and dyslipidaemia, are also very commonly present in association with diabetes. A patient with type 2 diabetes has a 2–4-fold increased risk of ischaemic heart disease resulting in angina and myocardial infarction, a 2–6-fold increased risk of stroke and a massively increased risk of peripheral vascular disease.

The above relates to accelerated atherosclerosis through abnormalities in lipid and lipoprotein metabolism, raised blood glucose leading to glycation of long-lived tissue proteins in the vasculature, adverse effects on the vascular endothelium, increased platelet interactions, and further acceleration by the common co-occurrence of hypertension and dyslipidaemia.

1.4.1 Clinical consequences in type 2 diabetes

The person with type 2 diabetes who has never had a vascular event is at the same risk of having an event as a non-diabetic person with a previous myocardial infarction (Haffner *et al.*, 1998) (Figure 1.4). If myocardial infarction occurs there is a significantly higher relative mortality (particularly in the younger age group) and increased likelihood of congestive heart failure compared with non-diabetes patients with a similar event (Singer *et al.*, 1989). The prognosis after

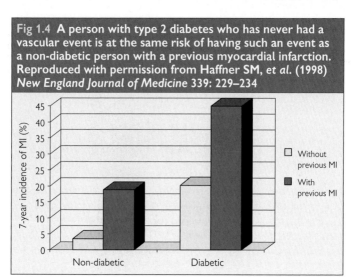

Fig 1.4 A person with type 2 diabetes who has never had a vascular event is at the same risk of having such an event as a non-diabetic person with a previous myocardial infarction. Reproduced with permission from Haffner SM, et al. (1998) *New England Journal of Medicine* 339: 229–234

myocardial infarction is significantly worse, perhaps related to more extensive atherosclerosis and increased rates of heart failure (Singer et al., 1989). The adverse effects of diabetes are particularly seen in women with loss of normal female protection (Pan et al., 1986). There is a significantly increased risk of stroke, which tends to leave more disability and is associated with higher mortality (Stamler et al., 1993). There is a greatly increased risk of peripheral vascular disease with intermittent claudication, rest pain, digital gangrene, increased propensity to infection and increased risk of lower limb amputation (Stamler et al., 1993) (Figure 1.5). The presence of proteinuria— either incipient (microalbuminuria) or overt (macroalbuminuria)—is associated with massively increased cardiovascular risk and mortality, i.e. renal protein leakage is not just something to do with the kidney but denotes generalized vascular damage/endothelial cell dysfunction (O'Donnell & Chowdhury, 2000).

In recent years a large evidence base has been built to inform on how best to manage the increased cardiovascular risk in diabetes patients; if properly applied, this can dramatically reduce both cardiovascular morbidity and mortality (see Chapter 3).

1.4.2 **Microvascular complications**
These cause significant morbidity and mortality, clinically apparent in the eyes, kidneys and nerves.

1.4.3 **Pathophysiology of diabetic microangiopathy**
This is a specific but generalized disorder of small blood vessels, i.e. specific to diabetes but generalized in that it can appear in virtually every small vessel in the body (Jennings & Barnett, 1988).

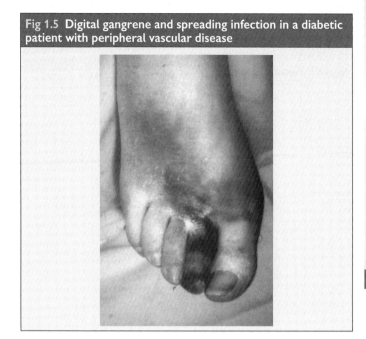

Fig 1.5 Digital gangrene and spreading infection in a diabetic patient with peripheral vascular disease

The histological hallmark is capillary basement membrane thickening in association with disruption of basement membrane architecture (Figure 1.6). This causes leakiness of plasma protein and profound abnormalities within the microcirculation.

The major risk factors for microvascular disease include the duration of diabetes and degree of metabolic control. The pathophysiology is not entirely understood but includes (Brownlee *et al.*, 1984; Jennings & Barnett, 1988):

- glycation of long-lived tissue proteins within capillary basement membrane
- haemostatic abnormalities
- functional abnormalities within the microcirculation
- deficiencies in redox state (with increased free radical production and reduced antioxidant levels)
- abnormalities of lipid metabolism
- hypertension
- genetic susceptibility.

All of the above may interact.

The fundamental pathology appears to be glycation of long-lived tissue proteins in capillary basement membrane. This results in the formation of advanced glycation end products, an irreversible

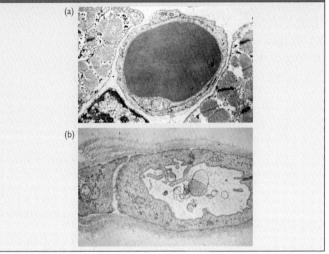

Fig 1.6 Electron micrographs of capillary (a) in cross-section with normal capillary basement membrane thickness, and (b) from a longstanding diabetic patient with thickened and abnormal basement membrane that leaks plasma protein

process, with continued accumulation over time (Brownlee et al., 1984). This leads to the basement membrane abnormalities discussed. Increased free radical production, endothelial cell dysfunction and increased platelet aggregation are also well reported. Lipid, haemostatic and prostaglandin abnormalities/imbalance lead to further endothelial cell damage and increased thrombotic tendency.

The above is compounded by hypertension which is present in around 80% of all patients with type 2 diabetes and is almost always present in association with significant microangiopathy.

1.5 Diabetic retinopathy

This is the commonest cause of blindness in the working population in the UK and many Western countries (Klein et al., 1998; Broadbent et al., 1999). Major susceptibility factors include disease duration and poor diabetes control, the latter leading to the changes in retinal microvasculature already described. Other ocular complications include cataract and other retinovascular diseases such as retinal vein occlusion, retinal artery occlusion and ischaemic optic atrophy. Glaucoma also occurs in at least 1% of the diabetes population. Age-related macular degeneration is also a major cause of severe visual impairment, particularly in the older population.

In the context of retinopathy development, increased blood flow in capillaries occurs due to a loss of pericytes in the normal retina causing disruption of retinal blood flow autoregulation (Donaldson & Dodson, 2003). Increased blood flow stimulates the production of vasoactive substances from the capillary wall and increasing endothelial cell proliferation eventually results in closure of the capillary circulation. This leads to retinal ischaemia with increased levels of growth factors which contribute to the pathology.

1.5.1 Stages of retinopathy

The stage of retinopathy are categorized in four groups.

1.5.1.1 Background retinopathy

This is common even at diagnosis of type 2 diabetes and includes microaneurysms, dot retinal haemorrhages and hard exudates without visual deterioration (Figure 1.7).

1.5.1.2 Maculopathy

These are retinal changes in the macular region, including ring-shaped exudates. Ischaemic maculopathy due to capillary closure within the macular area or a mixed form of the two may also occur. Maculopathy is the most common cause of diabetes blindness (Figure 1.8).

1.5.1.3 Preproliferative retinopathy

This may include cotton wool spots (areas of retinal ischaemia/infarction), venous abnormalities, arteriolar abnormalities and intraretinal microvascular abnormalities (Figure 1.9). These changes are highly predictive of the development of proliferative retinopathy within 2 years.

1.5.1.4 Proliferative retinopathy

This indicates severe ischaemia of the retina leading to new vessel formation in the optic disc or in the periphery of the retina or iris (Figure 1.10). Untreated, this can cause visual loss or blindness. New vessels may be asymptomatic until they rupture leading to pre-retinal, subhyaloid or vitreous haemorrhage (Figure 1.11).

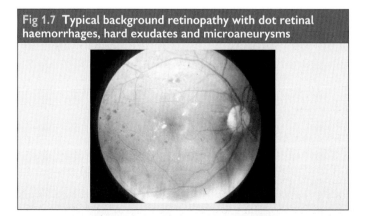

Fig 1.7 Typical background retinopathy with dot retinal haemorrhages, hard exudates and microaneurysms

Fig 1.8 Hard exudates coalescing around the macula and suggestive of maculopathy which can cause visual deterioration and blindness

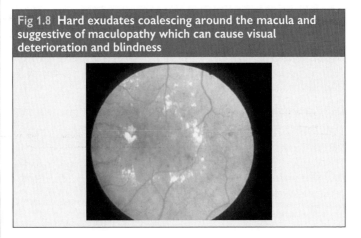

Fig 1.9 Preproliferative retinopathy with soft exudates and venous and arteriolar abnormalities

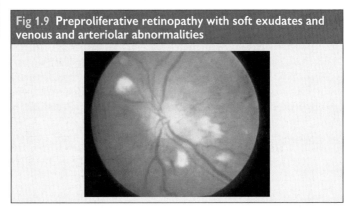

Fig 1.10 Proliferative retinopathy with new vessels in the disc, which are very liable to bleed thus causing blindness

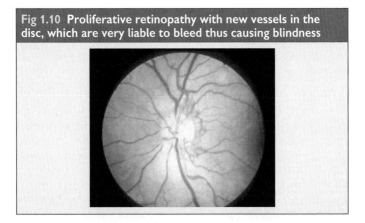

Fig 1.11 End-stage diabetic retinopathy with massive vitreous haemorrhage and retinal detachment causing blindness

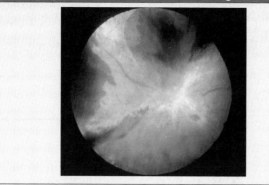

1.5.2 **Screening for diabetic retinopathy**

Digital photography is the method of choice in the UK; it produces good images with excellent sensitivity and specificity, and allows for quality assurance (UK National Screening Committee, 2004). It is extremely cost-effective coupled with appropriate treatment.

Laser treatment for maculopathy is given as focal or grid treatment depending on the site and degree of macular oedema. New vessel formation should be treated as an emergency by panretinal photocoagulation. This consists of multiple laser burns applied to the peripheral retina and can be extremely effective. Other interventions include vitrectomy with removal of the vitreous, dissection of new vessels and vitreoretinal traction, and application of laser treatment by endophotocoagulation.

Medical therapies have an important role in prevention and possibly treatment, and include a tight control of blood pressure and glycaemia (Donaldson & Dodson, 2003). There is preliminary evidence that angiotensin-converting enzyme (ACE) inhibitors or angiotensin receptor blockers might slow/prevent retinopathy, but definitive studies are awaited.

1.6 **Diabetic nephropathy**

The finding of protein leakage (normally in association with hypertension) heralds a massively increased risk of cardiovascular morbidity and mortality (Figure 1.12), together with an increased risk of the later development of frank renal failure and need for dialysis (Jarrett & Alberti, 1984; MacLeod et al., 1995). Around a quarter of people will show evidence of diabetic kidney disease, and the great increase in prevalence of type 2 diabetes in recent years means these patients have now overtaken those with type 1 diabetes in numbers of cases of chronic

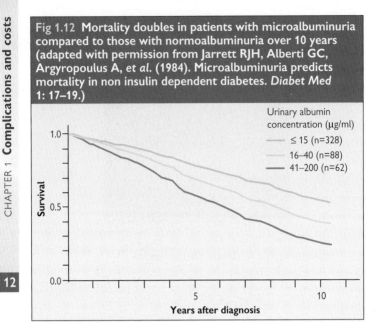

Fig 1.12 **Mortality doubles in patients with microalbuminuria compared to those with normoalbuminuria over 10 years (adapted with permission from Jarrett RJH, Alberti GC, Argyropoulus A, et al. (1984). Microalbuminuria predicts mortality in non insulin dependent diabetes. *Diabet Med* 1: 17–19.)**

renal failure. Diabetes is now the single commonest cause of chronic renal failure and need for dialysis in the UK and many other countries.

It is possible to identify the earliest stages of nephropathy by measuring the albumin excretion rate (AER) to identify microalbuminuria ('incipient' nephropathy), i.e. an AER above the normal range but below the level of standard 'dip stick' detection (Adler et al., 2003; Ritz, 2003). This strongly predicts later development of overt diabetic nephropathy and is associated with significantly increased cardiovascular risk.

Microalbuminuria is found in between 20% and 40% of all type 2 diabetic patients and is often found (as is overt macroproteinuria) even at diagnosis (Adler et al., 2003; Ritz, 2003).

1.6.1 **Natural history**

The major risk factors for nephropathy include duration of diabetes, poor metabolic control, and hypertension (Barnett, 2005). Others include cigarette smoking, certain forms of dyslipidaemia and protein overload.

Diabetic glomerulosclerosis is the microscopic description of diabetes nephropathy with a loss of normal histological architecture and the presence of glomerular basement membrane thickening (Figure 1.13). Both metabolic and haemodynamic factors are believed to be involved in its development and these include proteinuria commonly followed by reduction in glomerular filtration rate (GFR), glycation of long-lived tissue proteins and an increase in various growth factors.

Fig 1.13 (a) Normal glomerular architecture (H&E stain). (b) Diabetic glomerulosclerosis with glomerular basement membrane thickening and loss of normal histological architecture (H&E stain)

(a)

(b)

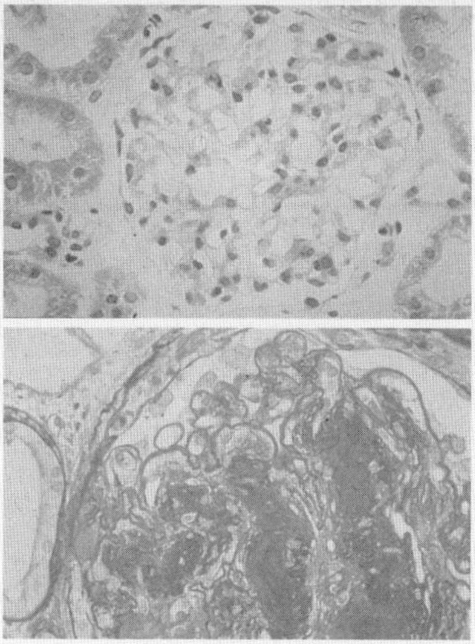

Even at diagnosis functional changes can be demonstrated within the diabetes kidney and are followed soon after by structural changes (Figure 1.14). The most important risk factor for progression and

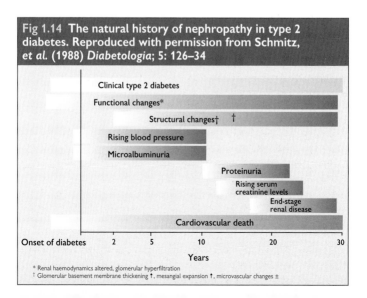

Fig 1.14 The natural history of nephropathy in type 2 diabetes. Reproduced with permission from Schmitz, et al. (1988) *Diabetologia*; 5: 126–34

Clinical type 2 diabetes

Functional changes*

Structural changes† †

Rising blood pressure

Microalbuminuria

Proteinuria

Rising serum creatinine levels

End-stage renal disease

Cardiovascular death

Onset of diabetes   2   5   10   20   30

Years

* Renal haemodynamics altered, glomerular hyperfiltration
† Glomerular basement membrane thickening ↑, mesangial expansion ↑, microvascular changes ±

probably development of diabetes renal disease is hypertension, and indeed this is present in around 50% of newly diagnosed type 2 diabetes patients and around 80% of established subjects, including virtually all those with persistent proteinuria.

Significant numbers of patients with type 2 diabetes already show evidence of protein leakage at diagnosis, and without intervention 5–10% of these subjects will convert to macroproteinuria (overt nephropathy) annually (Adler et al., 2003; Ritz, 2003). Persistent proteinuria is followed by a rise in serum creatinine and a gradual reduction in GFR, with the eventual development of end-stage renal disease without intervention unless the patient dies (usually from cardiovascular disease) before this phase is reached. The association of type 2 diabetes with hypertension and proteinuria indicates a particularly malignant form of this condition.

1.6.2 Screening for diabetic nephropathy

Screening for microalbuminuria in patients with type 2 diabetes will identify individuals who are at extremely high cardiovascular risk and also those with an increased risk of later development of renal failure. Semi-quantitative dip stick tests for microalbuminuria are now available, which if positive should lead to a laboratory estimate. The simplest measure is to take a spot urine and ask the laboratory for an albumin to creatinine ratio, which if raised above 2.5 mg/mmol in men and 3.5 mg/mmol in women on two or more occasions, and in the absence of other causes such as urinary tract infection, will diagnose incipient nephropathy.

If proteinuria is confirmed, other investigations include:

- measurement of electrolytes
- estimated GFR
- full blood count if there is a raised creatinine or reduced GFR as these patients are often anaemic
- lipid profile
- electrocardiography (ECG)
- consider renal ultrasound.

1.6.3 Management of nephropathy

The most important risk factors for the development and progression of nephropathy include poor diabetes control and hypertension (Adler et al., 2003; Ritz, 2003; Barnett, 2005). There is an excellent evidence base for the benefits of tightened glycaemic control in reducing the incidence of diabetes kidney disease both in type 1 and type 2 diabetes (Diabetes Control and Complications Trial Research Group, 1993; UKPDS Group, 1998a).

The evidence is also very good for blood pressure lowering, and indeed this is the most important aspect of management (Jarrett &

Alberti, 1984; MacLeod et al., 1995; Galr et al., 1997; Remuzzi et al., 2002; Adler et al., 2003; Ritz, 2003; Barnett, 2005). Systemic hypertension is normally accompanied by raised intraglomerular pressure in patients with nephropathy and this may relate to over-activation of the renin angiotensin system. The UK Prospective Diabetes Study (UKPDS) showed clearly the benefits of improving blood pressure (UKPDS Group, 1998b). There is particularly good evidence that drugs which inhibit the renin angiotensin system (i.e. ACE inhibitors and angiotensin II receptor blockers) will not only benefit diabetes kidney disease from the point of view of systemic blood pressure lowering, but may also have specific effects on the renal microcirculation by reducing raised intraglomerular pressure, thereby protecting the kidney. These effects have been shown at all stages of diabetes kidney disease (Brenner et al., 2001; Lewis et al., 2001; Parving et al., 2001; Barnett et al., 2004; ADVANCE Collaborative Group 2007), including prevention (Ruggenenti et al., 2004).

The most important point, however, is that very tight blood pressure control is vital (ideally less than 130/80) by whatever means necessary, but the regime used should normally include an inhibitor of the renin angiotensin system. In addition, use of other cardiopro-tective drugs including a statin and possibly low dose aspirin (once blood pressure is controlled) are vital, together with advice on smoking cessation, weight management, physical activity and alcohol ingestion.

1.7 Diabetic neuropathy

This is the most common complication of diabetes and most patients with type 2 diabetes will show evidence of nerve conduction abnor-malities after 5 years.

There are many classifications and the following is the author's pragmatic division.

1.7.1 (Distal symmetrical) chronic sensory neuropathy

This is the commonest type and may present with reduced sensation or paraesthesia in the feet but is often totally asymptomatic. Both metabolic and microvascular factors appear to be involved in devel-opment and progression. Although the neuropathy is predominantly sensory in nature, there may be weakness in the small muscles of the foot, accounting in part for the characteristic clawing of the toes and abnormal stresses over weight-bearing areas such as the tops of the toes and the metatarsal heads. This will lead to a build up of callus in association with loss of sensation which leads to further damage. The callus builds up and tends to crack forming a pool of exudate

Fig 1.15 Development of a typical neuropathic ulcer over the metatarsal heads. The ulcer has had callus removed by a chiropodist

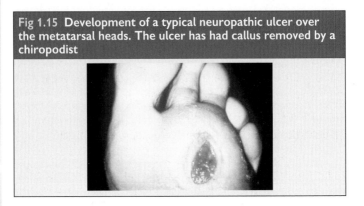

at the base of the crack, which will then commonly progress to development of a neuropathic ulcer over weight-bearing areas such as the metatarsal heads and tips of the toes (Figure 1.15). Infection may be a big problem in diabetes ulcers and may be localized or lead to cellulitis or even osteomyelitis.

Chronic sensory neuropathy may also be associated with the development of a Charcot joint due to a combination of localized osteoporosis and loss of sensation accompanied by (frequently minor) trauma. This may lead to inflammation in the joint and collapse—commonly the ankle or mid-tarsal joints (Figure 1.16). Appearances may initially mimic osteomyelitis, and if management is inappropriate there may be complete collapse of the joint with eventual bony ankylosis and loss of normal joint mobility leading to fixation and loss of function. Because of abnormal stresses in that area, neuropathic ulcers may develop in unusual places on the foot. Charcot arthropathy is commonly associated with recurrent infections of the foot and often the need for major amputation of the leg.

Fig 1.16 Charcot joint with loss of normal joint architecture, bony collapse and ankylosis with fixation of the joint and loss of function

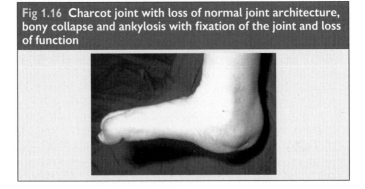

Screening for diabetes neuropathy is important and should always be part of the diabetes annual review. This should include:

- sensory testing for light touch and vibration sense
- ankle and knee reflexes
- evaluation of the condition of the feet and nails, including
  - examination for ulceration and skin breaks
  - general advice about foot care.

If ulceration develops it will require multiprofessional care.

1.7.2 Autonomic neuropathy

This is commonly found in association with chronic sensory neuropathy and, if symptomatic, has a poor prognosis. Epidemiological data suggest approximately 50% of symptomatic patients die within 5 years, usually from cardiac or cardiorespiratory problems (Ewing et al., 1980), although nowadays with better methods for cardioprotection this may now be a significant overestimate.

Manifestations include bladder dysfunction, diarrhoea, gastroparesis, postural hypotension and resting tachycardia. Erectile dysfunction in men may also be associated but is more commonly the result of vascular disease and/or psychological problems. Autonomic neuropathy is difficult to manage and treatment is mainly symptomatic.

1.7.3 Acute diabetic neuritis

This is less common and may present with burning feet, shooting pains down the legs and development of mononeuritis involving the third or sixth cranial nerves or the median, ulnar or femoral nerves. Femoral neuropathy, in particular, can be a serious condition with gross weight loss accompanied by significant wasting and weakness of the quadricep muscles with loss of knee jerks (sometimes with preservation of ankle jerks). Complete recovery may occur over months or years.

The acute neuropathies are often self-limiting but may require significant support as they can be very debilitating. Management involves tight diabetes control and analgesics, together with more specific treatments depending on symptoms.

1.8 Foot problems in the diabetic patient

Foot problems in diabetes may result from chronic sensory neuropathy, autonomic neuropathy and peripheral vascular disease. The latter is very common in people with type 2 diabetes and results from accelerated atherogenesis. It may present with intermittent claudication or even rest pain, and even mild trauma can lead to arterial ulceration and digital gangrene. Infection may arise from ulcers or elsewhere in the foot or leg and may include cellulitus, osteomyelitis and extensive gangrene. Patients with peripheral vascular disease commonly have disease in other vascular beds and the major cause of death in these patients is cardiac.

Management of diabetic foot problems involves a multiprofessional team to focus on prevention, including advice on foot hygiene, attention to the health of the nails, fitting appropriate shoes for high risk feet and regular visits to the chiropodist. Patients should be advised to immediately report any breaks in the skin or signs of infection or ulceration. If foot ulceration occurs, management involves elevation of the limb, appropriate antibiotics, good diabetes control (normally requiring insulin) and appropriate dressings.

1.9 **Costs of diabetes complications**

Diabetes now accounts for around 10% of the total healthcare budget of the UK (projections indicate that this could be as high as 25% within 20 years). The vast majority of these costs (around 80%) are a direct result of long-term complications, arising from cardiovascular care and managing blindness, visual deterioration, renal failure (including dialysis—cost £300 million per year in the UK) and limb amputation (Songer, 1992; American Diabetes Association, 1993; British Diabetic Association, 1995; Currie et al., 1997; Baxter et al., 2000).

The expenses incurred in the treatment of long-term complications far exceed the cost of drug therapies to prevent/ameliorate these. The latter are aimed at reducing risk by controlling factors such as lipids, glycaemia and blood pressure. Indeed, it is false economy to withhold effective intervention from patients with type 2 diabetes in the hope of saving money. Complications will always win!

1.10 **Conclusion**

Although the epidemic of type 2 diabetes is extremely serious and numbers of cases are increasing dramatically, it is the long-term complications that account for the vast majority of morbidity, mortality and cost. Complications can be divided into cardiovascular (which may result in coronary artery disease, stroke and peripheral vascular disease) and small vessel (microangiopathic) disease resulting in development of eye, kidney and nerve damage leading to blindness, renal failure and amputation. We now understand something of the pathophysiology involved in the development of diabetes vascular disease and have a good evidence base for treatment. Enaction of this knowledge presents a great challenge to health professionals and their patients and will involve adequate organization of care, overcoming concordance issues and the use of evidence-based therapies including lifestyle advice (see Chapter 8).

References

Adler AI, Stevens RJ, Manley SE, et al. (2003) Development and progression of nephropathy in type 2 diabetes: the United Kingdom Prospective, Diabetes Study (UKPDS 64). *Kidney Int* **63**: 225–32.

ADVANCE Collaborative Group (2007) Effects of a fixed combination of perindopril and indapamide on macrovascular and microvascular outcomes in patients with type 2 diabetes mellitus (the ADVANCE trial): a randomised controlled trial. *Lancet* **370**: 829–40.

American Diabetes Association (1993) *Direct and Indirect Costs of Diabetes in the USA in 1992.* American Diabetes Association, Alexandria, VA.

Barnett AH (2005). Pathogenesis and natural history. In: Barnett A (ed.) *Diabetes and Renal Disease*, pp. 17–22. Medical Education Partership Ltd., London.

Barnett AH, Bain SC, Bouter P, et al. (2004) Diabetics Exposed to Telmisartan and Enalapril Study Group. Angiotensin-receptor blockade versus converting-enzyme inhibition in type 2 diabetes and nephropathy. *N Engl J Med* **351**: 1952–61.

Barnett AH, Dixon AN, Bellary S, Hanif MW, O'Hare JP, Raymond NT, Kumar S (2006) Type 2 diabetes and cardiovascular risk in the UK South Asian community. *Diabetologia* **49**: 2234–46.

Barnett AH, O'Gara G, (eds) (2004) *Diabetes and Cardiovascular Disease* Medical Education Partership Ltd., London.

Baxter H, Bottomley J, Burns E, et al. (2000) CODE-2 UK: the annual direct costs of care for people with type 2 diabetes in the UK. *Diabet Med* **17**: 13.

Brenner BM, Cooper ME, de Zeeuw D, et al. (2001) RENAAL Study investigators. Effect of losartan on renal and cardiovascular outcomes in patients with type 2 diabetes and nephropathy. *N Engl J Med* **345**: 861–9.

British Diabetic Association (1995) *Diabetes in the UK—1996.* British Diabetic Association, London.

Broadbent DEM, Scott JA, Vora JP, et al. (1999) Prevalence of diabetic eye disease in an inner city population: the Liverpool Diabetic Eye Study. *Eye* **13**: 160–5.

Brownlee M, Vlassara H. Cerami A (1984) Non-enzymatic glycosylation and the pathogenesis of diabetic complications. *Ann Intern Med* **101**: 527–37.

Currie CJ, Kraus D, Morgan CL, et al. (1997) NHS acute sector expenditure for diabetes: the present, future and excess in-patient cost of care. *Diabet Med* **14**: 686–92.

Despres JP, Lemieux I, Prud'homme D (2001) Treatment of obesity: need to focus on high risk abdominally obese patients. *BMJ* **322**: 716–20.

Diabetes Control and Complications Trial Research Group (1993) The effect of intensive treatment of diabetes on the development and progression of long-term complications in insulin-dependent diabetes mellitus. *N Engl J Med* **329**: 977–86.

Donaldson M, Dodson PM (2003) Medical treatment of diabetic retinopathy. *Eye* **17**: 550–62.

Ewing DJ, Campbell IW, Clarke BNF (1980) The natural history of diabetic autonomic neuropathy. *QJ Med* **193**: 95–108.

Ford ES, Giles WH, Dietz WH (2002) Prevalence of the metabolic syndrome among US adults: findings from the third National Health and Nutrition Examination Survey. *JAMA* **287**: 356–9.

Gall MA, Hougaard P, Borch-Johnsen K, *et al.* (1997) Risk factors for development of incipient and overt diabetic nephropathy in patients with non-insulin dependent diabetes mellitus: prospective, observational study. *BMJ* **314**: 783–8.

Haffner SM, Lehto S, Ronnemaa T, *et al.* (1998) Mortality from coronary heart disease in subjects with type 2 diabetes and in non-diabetic subjects with and without prior myocardial infarction. *N Engl J Med* **339**: 229–34.

IDF (International Diabetes Federation) (2005) The IDF Consensus Worldwide Definition of the Metabolic Syndrome. Brussels IDF. Available from www.idf.org/webdata/docs/IDF, metasyndrome definition pdf (accessed November 2005).

Jarrett RJH, Alberti GC, Argyropoulus A, *et al.* (1984) Microalbuminuria predicts mortality in non insulin dependent diabetes. *Diabet Med* **1**: 17–19.

Jennings PE, Barnett AH (1988) New approaches to the pathogenesis and treatment of diabetic microangiopathy. *Diabet Med* **5**: 111–17.

Jensen MD, Haymond MW, Rizza RA, *et al.* (1989) Influence of body fat distribution on free fatty acid metabolism in obesity. *J Clin Invest* **83**: 1168–73.

Klein R, Klein BE, Moss SE, *et al.* (1998) The Wisconsin Epidemiologic Study of Diabetic Retinopathy: XVII. The 14-year incidence and progression of diabetic retinopathy and associated risk factors in type 1 diabetes. *Ophthalmology* **105**: 1801–15.

Lewis EJ, Hunsicker LG, Clarke WR, *et al.* (2001) Collaborative Study Group. Renoprotective effect of the angiotensin-receptor antagonist irbesartan in patients with nephropathy due to type 2 diabetes. *N Engl J Med* **345**: 851–60.

MacLeod JM, Lutale J, Marshall SM (1995) Albumin excretion and vascular deaths in NIDDM. *Diabetologia* **38**: 610–16.

McTernan P, Kumar S (2004) Pathogenesis of obesity-related type 2 diabetes. In: AH Barnett, S Kumar S (eds) *Obesity and Diabetes*, pp. 49–78. John Wiley & Sons, Chichester.

National Cholesterol Education Program (2002) Third Report of the Expert Panel on Detection, Evaluation and Treatment of High Blood Cholesterol in Adults (Adult Treatment Panel III). National Institute of Health, Bethesda, MD.

O'Donnell MJ, Chowdhury TA (2000) Hypertension and nephropathy in diabetes. In: AH Barnett, PM Dodson (eds) *Hypertension and Diabetes*, 3rd edn, pp. 21–31. Science Press Ltd, London.

Pan WH, Cedres LB, Liu K, *et al.* (1986) Relationship of clinical diabetes and asymptomatic hyperglycemia to risk of coronary heart disease mortality in men and women. *Am J Epidemiol* **123**: 504–16.

Parving H-H, Lehnert H, Brochner-Mortensen J, *et al.* (2001) Irbesartan in Patients with Type 2 Diabetes and Microalbuminuria Study Group. The effect of irbesartan on the development of diabetic nephropathy in patients with type 2 diabetes. *N Engl J Med* **345**: 870–8.

Reaven GM (1988) Banting Lecture 1988. Role of insulin resistance in human disease. *Diabetes* **37**: 1595–607.

Remuzzi G, Schieppati A, Ruggenenti P (2002) Nephropathy in patients with type 2 diabetes. *N Engl J Med* **346**: 1145–51.

Ritz E (2003) Albuminuria and vascular damage—the vicious twins. *N Engl J Med* **348**: 2349–52.

Ruggenenti P, Fassi A, Ilieva AP, *et al.* (2004) Preventing microalbuminuria in type 2 diabetes. *N Engl J Med* **351**: 1941–51.

Singer DE, Moulton AW, Nathan DM (1989) Diabetic myocardial infarction. Interaction of diabetes with other preinfarction risk factors. *Diabetes* **38**: 350–57.

Songer T (1992) The economic costs of NIDDM. *Diabet Metab Rev* **8**: 389–404.

Stamler J, Vaccaro O, Neaton JD, Wentworth D (1993) Diabetes, other risk factors and 12-year mortality for mean as screened in the multiple risk factor intervention trial. *Diabet Care* **16**: 434–44.

UK National Screening Committee (2004) *Essential Elements in Developing a Diabetic Retinopathy Screening Programme.* UK National Screening Committee, London. www.nscretinopathy.org.uk (epub).

UKPDS (UK Prospective Diabetes Study) Group (1998a) Intensive blood glucose control with sulphonyulureas or insulin compared with conventional treatment and risk of complications in patients with type 2 diabetes (UKPDS 33). *Lancet* **352**: 837–53.

UKPDS (UK Prospective Diabetes Study) Group (1998b) Tight blood pressure control and risk of macrovascular and microvascular complications in type 2 diabetes: UKPDS 38. *BMJ* **317**: 703–13.

WHO (World Health Organization) (1999) Definition, Diagnosis and Classification of Diabetes Mellitus and its Complications. Part 1. Diagnosis and classification of diabetes mellitus. World Health Organization, Geneva.

Yusuf S, Hawken S, Ounpuu S, *et al.* (2004) INTERHEART Study Investigators. Effect of potentially modifiable risk factors associated with myocardial infarction in 52 countries (the INTERHEART study): case-control study. *Lancet* **364**: 937–52.

Chapter 2

Pathophysiology of type 2 diabetes

Sarah Steven and Roy Taylor

Key points

- There are defects in both insulin sensitivity and insulin secretion
- Environmental factors determine prevalence in populations and risk in individuals
- Longstanding positive energy balance is a *sine qua non* of type 2 diabetes
- Liver fat levels are elevated before onset of type 2 diabetes
- Genetic factors determine degree of susceptibility to environmental influences
- Even extreme degrees of insulin resistance do not cause hyperglycaemia if beta cell function is good
- Decrease in beta cell function characterizes the transition from impaired glucose tolerance to diabetes
- Excess deposition and availability of fat within organs, particularly the liver, is central in the pathophysiology of type 2 diabetes.

2.1 Overview

Type 2 diabetes is preceded by insulin resistance usually of many years' duration. Onset is determined by loss of ability of beta cells to respond acutely to an increase in plasma glucose. The underlying factors which link these phenomena are becoming clearer. Although type 2 diabetes predominantly affects the overweight or obese it is clear that individuals vary in susceptibility: most morbidly obese people do not have diabetes, yet some modestly overweight people develop the condition. However, as a population becomes affluent and the prevalence of obesity increases, the incidence of type 2 diabetes rises sharply. These simple observations allow confident deduction that environmental factors have a dominant influence as the prevalence can change dramatically over one or two generations. On the other hand genetic factors are likely to explain why individuals with identical environmental risk exposure may or may not develop the condition.

2.2 Maintenance of glucose homeostasis

Euglycaemia is maintained by a balance between the appearance of glucose in the circulation and the uptake of glucose by tissues. It is imperative that plasma glucose is tightly regulated to protect cells from hyperglycaemia yet ensure continuous supply for tissues which depend upon glucose. Hence, the body must be able to adapt to periods of fasting as well as to sudden intake of food. These two states will be considered separately.

2.2.1 **Fasting state**

During an overnight fast, plasma glucose must be kept at levels which will ensure sufficient supply for the brain. The rate of flux through the plasma glucose pool is rapid, involving complete turnover of all glucose molecules within around one and a half hours. The steady plasma glucose level is best imagined as the level of water in a bath with plug out and taps full on. If the main regulator (insulin) turns down the taps, the level will fall. Only small changes of insulin concentration are required for this, far below the levels needed to affect uptake of glucose by other tissues. It can be seen that the overnight plasma insulin level will determine fasting plasma glucose.

Production of glucose by the liver depends on two processes. During the first 8–12 hours of fasting, plasma glucose is maintained mainly by breakdown of hepatic glycogen stores, a process inhibited by insulin and facilitated by glucagon. Gradually gluconeogenesis becomes the major process. This depends upon the 3-carbon compounds lactate, pyruvate, alanine and glycerol. During fasting there is a controlled mobilization of fat stores and an increase in non-esterified fatty acid levels (NEFA).

2.2.2 **Post-prandial state**

The immediate metabolic consequence of eating is suppression of hepatic glucose output as plasma insulin levels begin to rise, and in healthy people the liver has stopped exporting glucose within 30 minutes. Glucose uptake into muscle and liver is stimulated, and glucose oxidation rises. Net storage of glucose as glycogen happens over several hours after a meal. Approximately 30% of meal carbohydrate is stored as muscle glycogen and 20% as liver glycogen in

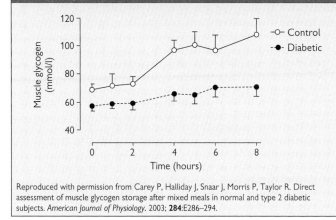

Fig 2.1 Change in muscle glycogen after eating breakfast (0 hours) and lunch (4 hours) in people with type 2 diabetes (closed circles) compared to those with normal glucose tolerance (open circles) as measured by ^{13}C magnetic resonance spectroscopy.

Reproduced with permission from Carey P, Halliday J, Snaar J, Morris P, Taylor R. Direct assessment of muscle glycogen storage after mixed meals in normal and type 2 diabetic subjects. *American Journal of Physiology*. 2003; **284**:E286–294.

healthy people 4 to 5 hours after eating. Lipolysis is suppressed in response to rising insulin levels and NEFA levels fall.

2.2.3 Differences in diabetes

In type 2 diabetes fasting hepatic glucose output is greater than normal, and as a consequence fasting blood glucose is elevated. This is so despite supra-normal plasma insulin levels, indicating that the liver is relatively resistant to insulin action.

After eating, both failure to suppress hepatic glucose output completely and failure of stimulation of storage of glucose as muscle glycogen (Figure 2.1) conspire to contribute to the elevated postprandial blood glucose typical of type 2 diabetes.

2.3 Insulin action and insulin resistance

The pathway of insulin signalling is now well understood. Insulin exerts its actions by binding to specific cell membrane receptors which are large transmembrane glycoproteins. The intra-cellular part of the receptor is a tyrosine kinase which triggers a known cascade of phosphorylation and dephosphorylation reactions. This leads to translocation of glucose transporters to the cell membrane increasing glucose uptake in muscle and adipose tissue; activation of the enzyme glycogen synthase; stimulation of phosphofructokinase and pyruvate dehydrogenase which regulate glycolysis and glucose oxidation respectively. However, there is no primary defect in the insulin signalling network in type 2 diabetes.

Insulin resistance is a key feature of type 2 diabetes. This is defined as the inability of insulin to produce its usual biological actions at any given concentration. Insulin action is usually measured solely in terms of glucose metabolism (and not other actions such as protein synthesis or ion transport across membranes). It is vital to understand that there are two levels of regulation in metabolism—substrate control and hormonal control. Competition between the main substrates—glucose and fat—is a very potent regulator. In normal subjects, raising the level of fatty acids in plasma will suppress glucose utilization by the process of substrate competition and by directly inhibiting glucose transport into muscle. In people with type 2 diabetes there are increases in plasma fatty acid levels as well as increased fat levels within the major metabolic organs (muscle and liver). Presence of excess fatty acids and metabolites such as diacylglycerol are the major factors producing what is described as 'insulin resistance'.

2.3.1 Lipotoxicity

The observation that fatty acids can impair glucose metabolism has been recognized for over 40 years. Randle hypothesized that elevated fatty acid concentrations inhibited several enzymes of the glycolytic pathway causing feedback inhibition of cellular glucose uptake. Recently magnetic resonance spectroscopy studies showed the main site of interaction between glucose and fat metabolism is at the level of glucose transport into the cell. In total lipodystrophy, there is no subcutaneous adipose tissue repository to store triglycerides. Although individuals with the condition look thin, they have high fat levels in muscle and liver and have extreme insulin resistance. This experiment of nature underscores the importance of Randle's observations.

Substrate competition as described above explains the insulin resistance associated with obesity, type 2 diabetes, lipodystrophy and ageing. Fatty acids have the most important interaction with glucose metabolism. Apart from the interaction at the level of glucose transport, other mechanisms appear to operate. When there is an imbalance between the supply of intracellular lipid and the cells capacity to utilize it, either by oxidation or by storage as metabolically inert triglyceride, there is an abnormal accumulation of intracellular diacylglycerol. Increased diacylglycerol activates novel protein kinase C and subsequently impairs insulin action. In normal circumstances, diacylglycerol is converted to triglyceride and the tissues are protected from fat-induced insulin resistance. However, when the supply of fatty acids exceeds the capacity of cells to oxidize or store fat as triglyceride, glucose metabolism is impaired.

Although obesity is a major predictor of type 2 diabetes there is clearly a high degree of inter-individual variation in its effect on insulin sensitivity. Only about 50% of people with a body mass index of more than 40 kg/m^2 will develop diabetes. Further work is required to establish why some obese individuals remain metabolically normal and are protected from the deleterious effects of excess fatty acids. An increased capacity of adipocytes to store metabolically inactive triacylglycerol in these individuals has been postulated as one mechanism.

2.3.2 Liver

Resistance of the liver to the effects of insulin (hepatic insulin resistance) in type 2 diabetes results in a failure of insulin to suppress hepatic glucose production. There is unsuppressed glycogenolysis and gluconeogenesis. As well as being the major determinant of fasting hyperglycaemia, decreased sensitivity of the liver to insulin contributes to post-prandial hyperglycaemia. Uptake of glucose by hepatocytes, unlike muscle and fat cells, depends entirely on the extracellular concentration of glucose and is not regulated by insulin.

2.3.3 Muscle

Muscle insulin resistance results in impaired glucose uptake by skeletal muscle and decreased glycogen storage. Figure 2.1 illustrates that fasting muscle glycogen concentration is subnormal, and that the impaired synthesis of glycogen in muscle over the hours following meals is severely impaired in people with type 2 diabetes. The failure to store glucose derived from ingested carbohydrate is striking, especially so when it is considered that the concentration of plasma insulin after the second meal was two and a half times greater than in the normal subjects. Skeletal muscle is a large organ (20 kg in the average man). As the glucose is not stored in muscle it remains in plasma, resulting in the marked post-prandial hyperglycaemia.

2.3.4 Adipose tissue

Resistance of adipose tissue to the effects of insulin results in inadequate suppression of lipolysis and modestly increased non-esterified fatty acid levels. Cytokines produced by adipose tissue such as resistin and adiponectin may help with fine regulation of metabolism. Secretion of TNF-α plays no part in the pathogenesis of type 2 diabetes.

2.4 Genetic and environmental factors contributing to insulin resistance

2.4.1 Obesity

The prevalence of type 2 diabetes in a population is reflected by the prevalence of obesity. A European study found that weight gain, measured as the change in BMI, in men and women in early adult-hood (25–40 years of age) was more strongly associated with risk of type 2 diabetes than was a subsequent increase in BMI. Also, greater weight gain, particularly in early adulthood, resulted in a younger age at onset of diabetes. One potential confounder is that BMI is a relatively insensitive marker as it does not reflect body composition, fat mass being important in terms of insulin sensitivity. Moreover it has been recognized for some time that fat distribution as well as fat mass is key with android fat pattern ('apple-shaped') being associated with insulin resistance and gynaecoid pattern ('pear-shaped') being protective. This is thought to be due to increased metabolic activity of visceral adipo-cytes compared to subcutaneous adipocytes. Visceral adipocytes are less responsive to suppression of lipolysis by insulin and more sensitive to lipolysis induced by catecholamines. The result could be increased delivery of free fatty acids to the liver through the portal circulation.

2.4.2 **Fatty liver**

It is now clear that fat accumulation within organs is important in the pathophysiology of type 2 diabetes. Liver fat content is pro-portional to obesity and inversely proportional to physical activity levels. In individuals with type 2 diabetes, the sensitivity of the liver to the effects of insulin is closely correlated with liver fat content and similarly skeletal muscle insulin sensitivity is related to intramyo-cellular fat content. Fat accumulation in the liver has been shown, independently of body mass and obesity, to be related to fasting hyperinsulinaemia, hypertriglyceridaemia and lower suppression of endogenous glucose production by insulin.

Type 2 diabetes is strongly associated with non-alcoholic fatty liver disease, a spectrum of liver damage which ranges from minor steato-sis to non-alcoholic steatohepatitis. The best available evidence sug-gests that excess liver fat deposition in the liver is uniformly present before the onset of classical type 2 diabetes. A prospective study of 3,189 Japanese workers aged over 40 taking less than 20 g of alcohol per day has provided a unique insight. The subjects were classified into two groups according to liver fat levels on abdominal ultra-sonography and were followed up with regular 75 g oral glucose tolerance tests to detect the development of diabetes. In the group with fatty liver at baseline the incidence was almost 5 times that of those with normal liver fat after 8 years. The cumulative incidence of diabetes according to liver fat content is shown in Figure 2.2. This suggests that excess fat in the liver is an early and necessary step in the pathogenesis of type 2 diabetes.

In the liver, increased local and plasma-derived fatty acids result in increased production of VLDL-apolipoprotein B by the liver. This results in decreased HDL and increased small LDL particles, the latter being highly atherogenic. In addition, the fatty liver overproduces

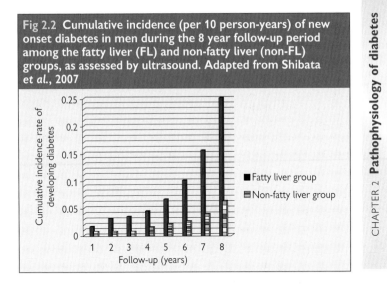

Fig 2.2 **Cumulative incidence (per 10 person-years) of new onset diabetes in men during the 8 year follow-up period among the fatty liver (FL) and non-fatty liver (non-FL) groups, as assessed by ultrasound. Adapted from Shibata** *et al.*, 2007

plasminogen activator inhibitor-1, coagulation factors and C-reactive protein. Together these abnormalities provide an explanation for the increased risk of cardiovascular disease in fatty liver disease and in type 2 diabetes in particular.

Although hepatic fat accumulation is strongly associated with decreased insulin sensitivity, a large variation exists between individuals. For the same degree of hepatic fat content individuals can be identified who have very high and very low insulin resistance. Recently the G allele variant of rs738409 in the *PNPLA3* gene (patatin like phospholipase-3) has been shown to be a genotype which seems to predispose to hepatic steatosis. Interestingly, this genotype is associated with liver damage but not with insulin resistance or unfavourable metabolic profile. The risk of metabolic disease may be able to be partially dissociated from the fatty liver disease risk; in some people hepatic steatosis is linked to obesity, dyslipidaemia and glucose intolerance and in others it is related to endogenous genetic predisposition to metabolically 'safe' liver fat accumulation.

2.4.3 **Physical activity**

The increasingly sedentary lifestyle of Western living is associated with earlier onset of type 2 diabetes. An 8 year follow-up study of 70,102 female nurses showed a progressive decrease in the relative risk of diabetes with increasing physical activity levels (Figure 2.3). There is substantial evidence that physical activity prevents or delays the onset of type 2 diabetes in those with impaired glucose tolerance. In the Diabetes Prevention Program, individuals with impaired

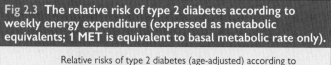

Fig 2.3 The relative risk of type 2 diabetes according to weekly energy expenditure (expressed as metabolic equivalents; 1 MET is equivalent to basal metabolic rate only).

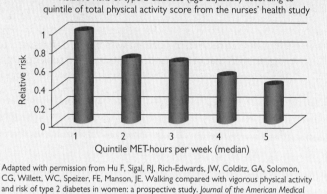

Relative risks of type 2 diabetes (age-adjusted) according to quintile of total physical activity score from the nurses' health study

Adapted with permission from Hu F, Sigal, RJ, Rich-Edwards, JW, Colditz, GA, Solomon, CG, Willett, WC, Speizer, FE, Manson, JE. Walking compared with vigorous physical activity and risk of type 2 diabetes in women: a prospective study. *Journal of the American Medical Association*. 1999;**282**:1433–1439.

glucose tolerance were randomized to placebo, metformin or a lifestyle programme involving 150 minutes of physical activity a week. After an average of 2.8 years of follow-up the lifestyle intervention was found to be superior to metformin in reducing the average incidence of diabetes; 11 compared to 7.8 cases per 100 person-years compared to 4.8 cases per 100 person-years in the placebo group. Physical activity has also been shown to improve glycaemic control and to reduce cardiovascular risk in those with established type 2 diabetes.

The mechanism for the beneficial effect of physical activity is mainly but not solely via improvement in fat handling between adipose tissue, liver and muscle and hence improvement in insulin sensitivity. Exercise specifically decreases liver fat content. Physical activity enhances GLUT4-dependent and hypoxia-dependent glucose transport in skeletal muscle and decreases plasma insulin levels.

2.4.4 **Genetic predisposition**

Single gene mutations represent a very small proportion of cases of diabetes (around 1%). However, a simple epidemiological observation highlights the importance of genetics in the development of type 2 diabetes: the prevalence of diabetes varies widely among diverse ethnic groups sharing a common environment. The Pima Indians of Arizona have the highest reported prevalence of type 2 diabetes mellitus (~40%) of any population in the world. This is so despite sharing a similar hypercaloric, sedentary environment with the wider US population (prevalence ~7%). The thrifty gene hypothesis suggests that in the past, times of famine caused selection pressures for a genotype that leads to efficient fat storage during times of abundance. Diabetes was unknown amongst the Pimas when they lived as subsistence farmers. In today's environment of constant exposure to positive calorie balance, their genotype is metabolically disadvantageous.

Family history is recognized to be particularly important in establishing an individual's risk of developing type 2 diabetes; the lifetime risk for a first-degree relative of a patient with type 2 diabetes is 5 to 10 times higher than that of age- and weight-matched subjects without a family history of diabetes. However, such observations cannot untangle the effect of genetics from the propensity for families to share similar eating patterns and physical activity levels.

A cross-sectional study using the population-based Danish Twin Register looked at prevalence, concordance rates and recurrence risks of type 2 diabetes and abnormal glucose tolerance in monozygotic and dizygotic twins. As monozygotic twins have identical genotypes, any differences are theoretically due to environmental factors. The probandwise concordance for type 2 diabetes was not significantly different (monozygotic 0.50 and dizygotic 0.37). For abnormal glucose tolerance there was a clearer separation (monozygotic 0.63 and dizygotic 0.43). This suggests that genetic predisposition might be important for the development of abnormal glucose tolerance, but that non-genetic factors may have a more important role determining whether a genetically predisposed subject progresses to overt type 2 diabetes. The concordance rate for abnormal glucose tolerance in dizygous twins in this study is interesting; it seems to be higher than the age-equivalent risk of type 2 diabetes of approximately 22% for first degree relatives. This suggests that there may be some important aspect of the twin status *per se*, such as sharing the same environment more closely or even sharing of the intrauterine environment.

2.4.5 Insights from bariatric surgery and hypocaloric dieting

The observation that bariatric surgery can reproducibly reverse type 2 diabetes is important in understanding the pathophysiology of the disease. This suggests that certainly up to some point beta-cell dysfunction is reversible. Of great significance is the observation that the restoration of normal fasting plasma glucose occurs before any significant weight has been lost. Figure 2.4 demonstrates the normalization of glucose levels within 7 days following bilio-pancreatic diversion. Euglycaemic-hyperinsulinaemic clamp studies have shown that within 7 days of gastric bypass surgery, insulin sensitivity doubles.

Normoglycaemia is regained in 99% of people with type 2 diabetes after biliopancreatic diversion, 84% after gastric bypass and 48% after gastric banding. The different effects of these procedures has been claimed to reflect the direct effect of the surgery upon

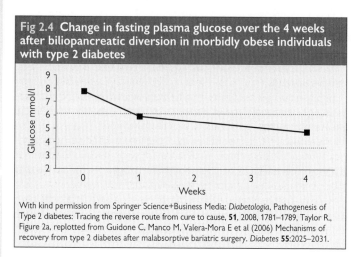

Fig 2.4 Change in fasting plasma glucose over the 4 weeks after biliopancreatic diversion in morbidly obese individuals with type 2 diabetes

With kind permission from Springer Science+Business Media: *Diabetologia*, Pathogenesis of Type 2 diabetes: Tracing the reverse route from cure to cause, **51**, 2008, 1781–1789, Taylor R., Figure 2a, replotted from Guidone C, Manco M, Valera-Mora E et al (2006) Mechanisms of recovery from type 2 diabetes after malabsorptive bariatric surgery. *Diabetes* **55**:2025–2031.

incretin hormone secretion. That is that exclusion of nutrients from the foregut and enhanced delivery of nutrients to the hindgut may enhance GLP-1 secretion and decrease GIP secretion thus improving insulin secretion. Despite this concept being widely accepted, the evidence on which these theories are based is inconsistent and diet alone is associated with changes in incretin secretion.

In clinical practice, it is occasionally noted that a particularly motivated person with type 2 diabetes can lose enough weight to normalize glucose levels. A study of weight loss in subjects with type 2 diabetes using hypocaloric diets rather than surgery has shown that after weight loss of 8 kg, fasting plasma glucose decreased markedly with an 81 +/– 4% decrease in intrahepatic lipid content. It follows that in both bariatric surgery and hypocaloric dieting, there is an early and rapid reduction in liver fat content which corresponds in time-course with the normalization of hepatic insulin sensitivity and normalization of fasting blood glucose. The mechanism for the early improvement in insulin secretion after biliopancreatic requires further investigation.

2.5 **Insulin secretion**

The release of insulin from beta-cells is coupled to ATP production due to increase in substrate supply. A rise in glucose availability within beta cells as plasma glucose levels begin to rise is the major trigger. Other substrates, notably amino acids, can also stimulate insulin release.

Glucose is transported into beta cells via GLUT2 receptors. It is then phosphorylated to glucose-6-phosphate with subsequent glycolysis and oxidation to produce adenosine triphosphate (ATP). ATP stimulates the closure of ATP-dependent cell membrane potassium channels, which depolarizes the cell membrane and results in an influx of calcium ions. Within beta-cells insulin is stored in secretory granules. In response to the rise in intracellular calcium levels, the secretory granules fuse with the cell membrane releasing insulin and C-peptide in equimolar amounts. In vivo approximately 50% of daily insulin production is released in a constant, pulsatile manner to achieve control of basal metabolism, with the remainder being released to control postprandial metabolism.

In response to a glucose stimulus/meal there is an acute increase in insulin release lasting about 10 minutes followed by a slower second phase of insulin release that can last for several hours. The initial acute rise in insulin can be defined as the first phase insulin response when the stimulus is intravenous glucose. The first phase response is thought to result from insulin released from secretory granules located near to the beta cell membrane. It is this early insulin response which suppresses endogenous glucose production at the start of a meal. In contrast, the second phase insulin response, evolves to ensure metabolic control during and after absorption of a meal. The abnormalities seen in insulin secretion in type 2 diabetes are listed in Box 2.1.

Two separate aspects of insulin secretion in diabetes must be clarified. Fasting hyperinsulinaemia reflects the failure of metabolic regulation with ambient high plasma glucose levels perpetuating this steady state. However, an acute increase in insulin after eating cannot be provided by the beta cells.

The defect in first phase insulin secretion is a characteristic feature in type 2 diabetes. Impairments in first phase insulin secretion may also serve as a marker of risk for type 2 diabetes mellitus in family members of individuals with type 2 diabetes mellitus and may be seen in patients with prior gestational diabetes. A study in a population of individuals with impaired glucose tolerance found that the absence of the peak of the first insulin secretion phase was the best predictor of incident type 2 diabetes.

Fatty acids are a fuel for beta-cells and when levels of fatty acids are acutely elevated insulin production is stimulated. Prolonged exposure

---

Box 2.1 The characteristic abnormalities of insulin secretion seen in type 2 diabetes

- Reduced or absent first-phase insulin response (Figure 2.5)
- Delayed responses to ingestion of meals
- Alterations in rapid pulses and oscillations of insulin secretion
- Defective beta cell proinsulin processing: increased circulating levels of plasma proinsulin and partially processed proinsulin molecules compared to insulin
- Reduced second phase insulin release
- Fasting hyperinsulinaemia.

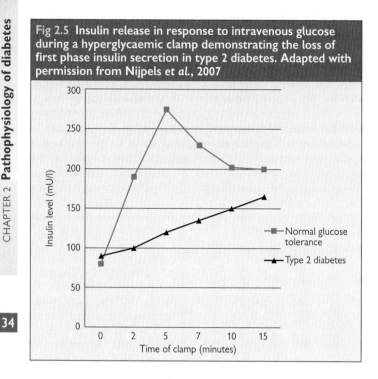

Fig 2.5 Insulin release in response to intravenous glucose during a hyperglycaemic clamp demonstrating the loss of first phase insulin secretion in type 2 diabetes. Adapted with permission from Nijpels *et al.*, 2007

of beta-cells to fatty acids increases basal insulin release but inhibits glucose-induced insulin secretion. This seems to relate to endoplasmic reticulum stress, mitochondrial dysfunction and initiation of apoptosis. Not all fatty acids are equal in their chronic action to inhibit glucose mediated insulin secretion. Saturated fatty acids are particularly potent, whereas monounsaturated fatty acids have actually been shown to have some protective effects upon beta-cells.

2.5.1 **Beta-cell mass**

Both defects in beta-cell mass and beta-cell function contribute to the pathophysiology of type 2 diabetes. The 80% decrease in insulin secretory capacity seen in hyperglycaemic clamp experiments in patients with type 2 diabetes cannot be solely caused by the reduction in beta-cell mass. It is evident that many patients undergoing pancreatic surgery can maintain normal glycaemic control after resection of large volumes of pancreatic tissue. Following hemipancreatectomy only 25% have abnormal glucose tolerance 1 year after surgery. Using fasting plasma glucose and insulin data beta-cell function is already reduced by about 50% at diagnosis of type 2 diabetes.

Studies of cadaveric pancreata have shown that beta cell mass is increased in obese individuals, but is deficient in both lean and obese individuals with type 2 diabetes. The question arises as to whether the defective beta-cell mass is caused by many years of diabetes, or whether it is a primary defect. The decline in beta-cell mass as type 2 diabetes progresses is likely to be exacerbated by the adverse metabolic environment for beta-cells.

Beta-cells turn over continuously during adult life, and cell numbers at any one time depend upon both apoptosis and generation of new cells. In type 2 diabetes, increased apoptosis has been demonstrated. In contrast, beta-cell replication and neogenesis (new islet formation from exocrine ducts) seems to be unaffected by type 2 diabetes. This understanding of the dynamics of the beta-cells explains why beta-cell mass can increase in adult life in the context of obesity and also during pregnancy. Increased islet cell replication can be enhanced in vitro with gastrin and other growth promoting factors. Targeting the mechanisms of beta-cell apoptosis and replication may proffer targets for future therapies for enhancing insulin secretion in type 2 diabetes.

2.5.2 Incretin action

There is a greater insulin response when a given amount of glucose is administered orally rather than intravenously and the presence of hormones originating from the intestine have long been postulated. More recently it has been suggested that an impaired incretin effect may contribute to beta-cell impairment in type 2 diabetes. Glucagon-like peptide 1 (GLP-1) and gastric inhibitory polypeptide (GIP) are incretin hormones which are released from the gut in response to eating. They augment insulin secretion by their effects on the beta cell. The GLP-1 response is blunted in type 2 diabetes and the beta-cell response to GIP is grossly impaired. Exogenous administration of GLP-1 in type 2 diabetes can result in near normal blood glucose. The effect can be exploited therapeutically by use of GLP-1 analogue injection or oral DPPIV which delay inactivation of endogenous GLP-1.

2.5.3 Islet cell amyloid

A frequently seen feature in islets of individuals with type 2 diabetes is amyloid deposition. Islet amyloid polypeptide (amylin) is co-secreted with insulin from beta cells. The available data regarding any pathogenic role for amylin in type 2 diabetes is far from convincing and it may be a secondary phenomenon resulting from dysregulated insulin secretion.

2.5.4 Lipotoxicity and the beta cell

Histological studies of the pancreas in classical type 2 diabetes consistently show 40–50% of normal numbers of beta cells, but they are not able to function normally. Beta-cells in vitro are unable to respond acutely to an increase in glucose concentration after exposure to increased fatty acid concentrations. In humans, a direct correlation has been demonstrated between beta cell triglyceride accumulation and rate of apoptosis. In obese rodents observed during the development of diabetes, the onset of hyperglycaemia is preceded by a rapid increase in pancreatic fat.

The fat content of the pancreas has been difficult to assess due to usual fixation methods. Specialized histological studies suggest a relationship between non-alcoholic fatty liver disease and pancreatic steatosis. Using novel magnetic resonance techniques it has been shown that pancreas fat levels are elevated in type 2 diabetes. The currently available information suggests that the type 2 diabetes defect in acute insulin secretion could be directly caused by excess fat around the beta-cells.

2.6 **Time course to development of type 2 diabetes**

Insulin resistance is the first identifiable abnormality in the development of type 2 diabetes. Beta-cell function steadily deteriorates during the progression from impaired glucose tolerance to overt type 2 diabetes. Data from UKPDS has been extrapolated in a linear fashion suggesting that beta-cell function has been steadily deteriorating for around 12 years. In contrast, direct observation of a large

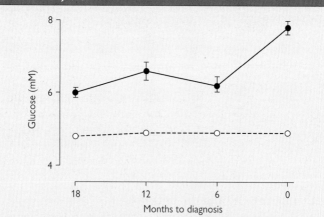

Fig 2.6 **In the West of Scotland Coronary Prevention Study fasting plasma glucose levels remain fairly constant until a few months prior to the diagnosis of diabetes. Data from Sattar et al., 2007**

With kind permission from Springer Science+Business Media: *Diabetologia*, Pathogenesis of Type 2 diabetes: Tracing the reverse route from cure to cause, **51**, 2008, 1781–1789, Taylor R., Figure 5a, replotted from Sattar N, McConnachie A, Ford I et al (2007) Serial metabolic measurements and conversion to type 2 diabetes in the West of Scotland Coronary Prevention Study: specific elevations in alanine aminotransferase and triglycerides suggest hepatic fat accumulation as a potential contributing factor. *Diabetes* **56**:984–991 group of subjects prospectively in the West of Scotland Coronary Prevention Study found that there was a very rapid increase in blood glucose levels in the 6 months preceding the diagnosis, rather than a steady upwards drift (Figure 2.6). The risk of incident diabetes was strongly associated with a sustained increase in plasma alanine amino-transferase levels, suggestive of steadily increasing accumulation of fat within the liver which places a burden on liver cells.

2.7 Current understanding of the pathophysiology of type 2 diabetes

By bringing together information on insulin sensitivity and insulin secretion with more recent knowledge on the deleterious effects of elevated fatty acids, the pathogenesis of type 2 diabetes can be described. Peripheral insulin resistance results in a compensatory increase in insulin secretion. Over time, hyperinsulinaemia in the portal circulation in combination with a positive calorie balance results in the accumulation of fat in the liver. Fatty liver results in a failure of insulin suppression of hepatic glucose output. Blood glucose levels rise, further exacerbating hyperinsulinaemia and increasing liver fat. This initiates a vicious cycle (Figure 2.7). The fatty liver overproduces VLDL and excess triglyceride is exported to all tissues including the pancreas. Excess fatty acids chronically suppresses glucose stimulated insulin production. At a threshold level which is individually determined, beta-cell decompensation occurs and blood glucose levels rise rapidly resulting in overt type 2 diabetes. This twin cycle hypothesis integrates recent observations with previously established metabolic information to explain aetiology and patho-genesis of type 2 diabetes.

Overall, positive energy balance over years is the essential factor in the development of fatty liver and eventually hyperglycaemia. Weight loss by diet or by bariatric surgery can reverse diabetes and this is associated with decrease in hepatic fat levels allowing recovery of insulin sensitivity. Decreased beta-cell apoptosis can be brought about in adult life by decreasing fatty acid availability. This new understanding of the pathophysiology of type 2 diabetes indicates need for a new approach to management.

Fig 2.7 **The Twin Cycle Hypothesis. Chronic energy intake that is in excess of requirements results in liver fat accumulation. As this process is promoted by insulin, individuals with a degree of insulin resistance will accumulate liver fat more readily than others. As the liver fat increases, hepatic glucose production becomes less sensitive to suppression by insulin, plasma glucose levels tend to rise and basal insulin secretion rate rises. This forms vicious cycle A (in dark blue). The increased liver fat will increase secretion of triacylglycerol from the liver. Pancreatic islets are susceptible to local triacylglycerol accumulation. The red arrows represent proximal steps to the onset of type 2 diabetes. The post-meal response to glucose becomes blunted, and this is exacerbated by the modestly raised plasma glucose. Vicious cycle B (in light blue) causes impaired glucose regulation, and eventually the fatty acid and glucose inhibitory effects on the islets reach a threshold, leading to a relatively sudden onset of clinical diabetes.**

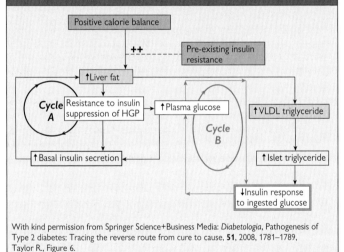

With kind permission from Springer Science+Business Media: *Diabetologia*, Pathogenesis of Type 2 diabetes: Tracing the reverse route from cure to cause, **51**, 2008, 1781–1789, Taylor R., Figure 6.

References

Balkau B, Mhamdi L, Oppert JM, *et al.* (2008) Physical activity and insulin sensitivity the RISC study. *Diabetes* **57**: 2613–18.

Butler A, Janson J, Bonner-Weir S, Ritzel R, Rizza R, Butler P (2003) Beta-cell deficit and increased beta-cell apoptosis in humans with type 2 diabetes. *Diabetes* **52**: 102–10.

Carey P, Halliday J, Snaar J, Morris P, Taylor R (2003) Direct assessment of muscle glycogen storage after mixed meals in normal and type 2 diabetic subjects. *Am J Physiol* **284**: E286–94.

Cnop M (2008) Fatty acids and glucolipotoxicity in the pathogenesis of Type 2 diabetes. *Biochem Soc Trans* **36**: 348–52.

Group DPPR (2002) Reduction in the incidence of type 2 diabetes with life-style intervention or metformin. *N Engl J Med* **346**: 393–403.

Guidone C, Manco M, Valera-Mora E, *et al.* (2006) Mechanisms of recovery from type 2 diabetes after malabsorptive bariatric surgery. *Diabetes* **55**: 2025–31.

Hanley S, Austin E, Assouline-Thomas B, *et al.* (2010) β-Cell mass dynamics and islet cell plasticity in human type 2 diabetes. *Endocrinology* **151**: 1462–72.

Hu F, Sigal RJ, Rich-Edwards JW, Colditz GA, Solomon CG, Willett WC, Speizer FE, Manson JE (1999) Walking compared with vigorous physical activity and risk of type 2 diabetes in women: a prospective study. *JAMA* **282**: 1433–9.

Johnson A, Argyraki M, Thow J, Cooper B, Fulcher G, Taylor R (1992) Effect of increased free fatty acid supply on glucose metabolism and skeletal muscle glycogen synthase activity in normal man. *Clinical Science* **82**: 219–26.

Kashyap S, Daud S, Kelly K, Gastaldelli A, Win H, Brethauer S, Kirwan J, Schauer P (2009) Acute effects of gastric bypass versus gastric restrictive surgery on beta-cell function and insulinotropic hormones in severely obese patients with type 2 diabetes. *Int J Obes (Lond)* **34**: 462–71.

Morgan N (2009) Fatty acids and beta-cell toxicity. *Curr Opin Clin Nutr Metab Care* **12**: 117–22.

Neel J (1962) Diabetes mellitus: a 'thrifty' genotype rendered detrimental by 'progress?'. *Am J Hum Genet* **14**: 353–62.

Nijpels G, Boorsma W, Dekker J, Hoeksema F, Kostense P, Bouter L, Heine R (2007) Absence of an acute insulin response predicts onset of Type 2 diabetes in a caucasian population with impaired glucose tolerance. *J Clin Endocrinol Metab* **93**: 2633–8.

Ofei F, Hurel S, Newkirk J, Sopwith M, Taylor R (1996) Effects of an engineered human anti-TNF alpha antibody (CDP571) on insulin sensitivity and glycemic control in patients with NIDDM. *Diabetes* **45**: 881–5.

Petersen K, Dufour S, Befroy D, Lehrke M, Hendler R, Shulman G (2005) Reversal of nonalcoholic hepatic steatosis, hepatic insulin resistance, and hyperglycemia by moderate weight reduction in patients with type 2 diabetes. *Diabetes* **54**: 603–8.

Roden M, Price T, Perseghin G, Petersen K, Rothman D, Cline G, Shulman G (1996) Mechanism of free fatty acid-induced insulin resistance in humans. *J Clin Invest* **97**: 2859–65.

Samuel V, Petersen K, Shulman G (2010) Lipid-induced insulin resistance: unravelling the mechanism. *Lancet* **375**: 2267–77.

Sattar N, McConnachie A, Ford I, *et al.* (2007) Serial metabolic measurements and conversion to type 2 diabetes in the west of Scotland coronary prevention study: specific elevations in alanine aminotransferase and triglycerides suggest hepatic fat accumulation as a potential contributing factor. *Diabetes* **56**: 984–91.

Schienkiewitz A, Schulze M, Hoffmann K, Kroke A, Boeing H (2006) Body mass index history and risk of type 2 diabetes: results from the European Prospective Investigation into Cancer and Nutrition (EPIC)–Potsdam Study. *Am J Clin Nutr* **84**: 427–33.

Seppala-Lindroos A, Vehkavaara S, Hakkinen A, *et al.* (2002) Fat accumulation in the liver is associated with defects in insulin suppression of glucose production and serum free fatty acids independent of obesity in normal men. *J Clin Endocrinol Metab* **87**: 3023–8.

Shibata M, Kihara Y, Taguchi M, Tashiro M, Otsuki M (2007) Nonalcoholic fatty liver disease is a risk factor for type 2 diabetes in middle-aged Japanese men. *Diabetes Care* **30**: 2940–4.

Shulman G, Rothman D, Jue T, Stein P, DeFronzo R, Shulman R (1990) Quantitation of muscle glycogen synthesis in normal subjects and subjects with non-insulin-dependent diabetes by 13C nuclear magnetic resonance spectroscopy [see comments] *N Engl J Med* **322**: 223–8.

Singhal P, Caumo A, Carey P, Cobelli C, Taylor R (2002) Regulation of endogenous glucose production after a mixed meal in type 2 diabetes. *Am J Physiol Endocrinol Metab* **283**: E275–83.

Speliotes E, Butler J, Palmer C, *et al.* (2010) PNPLA3 variants specifically confer increased risk for histologic nonalcoholic fatty liver disease but not metabolic disease. *Hepatology* **52**: 904–12.

Steven S, Lim EL, Taylor R (2010) Dietary reversal of Type 2 diabetes motivated by research knowledge. *Diabet Med* **27**: 724–5.

Taylor R (2008) Pathogenesis of Type 2 diabetes: Tracing the reverse route from cure to cause. *Diabetologia* **51**: 1781–9.

Taylor R, Magnusson I, Rothman D, Cline G, Caumo A, Cobelli C, Shulman G (1996) Direct assessment of liver glycogen storage by 13C nuclear magnetic resonance spectroscopy and regulation of glucose homeostasis after a mixed meal in normal subjects. *J Clin Invest* **97**: 126–32.

Taylor R, Price T, Katz L, Shulman, R, Shulman, G (1993) Direct measurement of change in muscle glycogen concentration after a mixed meal in normal subjects. *Am J Physiol* **265**: E224–9.

van der Heijden G, Wang Z, Chu Z, Sauer P, Haymond M, Rodriguez L, Sunehag A (2010) A 12-week aerobic exercise program reduces hepatic fat accumulation and insulin resistance in obese, Hispanic adolescents. *Obesity (Silver Spring)* **18**: 384–90.

Yki-Jarvinen H (2005) Fat in the liver and insulin resistance. *Ann Med* **37**: 347–56.

Chapter 3

Interpretation of recent clinical trials concerning tight glycaemic control and cardiovascular risk

Cristina Bianchi and Stefano Del Prato

> ### Key points
>
> Tight glycaemic control is still recommended by official guidelines, although:
>
> - Recent intervention trials have shown some impact on microvascular complications but limited or no effect on vascular risk
> - Microvascular benefit of tight glycaemic control should be weighed against the increase in total and CV-related mortality, increased weight gain, and risk for severe hypoglycaemia
> - Hypoglycaemia rather than a trigger factor for CV events may be a marker for vulnerable patients
> - Avoiding risks of tight glycaemic control requires
>   - Early and effective intervention
>   - Personalized glycaemic targets
>   - Careful selection of pharmacologic intervention.

3.1 Introduction

Type 2 diabetes (T2DM) is a chronic and progressive condition associated with the risk of invalidating micro- and macrovascular complications. Hyperglycaemia is the hallmark of the condition and a general consensus exists to suggest that treatment should aim at near-normoglycaemia. Several epidemiological studies have linked degree and duration of hyperglycaemia to the risk of developing long-term complications. However, we had to wait till the completion of the *United Kingdom Prospective Diabetes Study* (UKPDS) to have intervention data to support the value of appropriate glycaemic control in reducing the risk of long-term complications. Upon the publication of those landmark results the American Diabetes Association (ADA) emphatically stated that 'the results of the UKPDS mandate that treatment of type 2 diabetes includes aggressive efforts to lower blood glucose levels as close to normal as possible'. More recently, however, the foundation of this conviction has become less solid due to the results of recent intervention trials.

3.2 **Intervention trials in diabetes**

3.2.1 **The UKPDS and the Kumamoto study**
In the UKPDS, 3867 newly diagnosed T2DM patients were randomly assigned intensive policy with a sulfonylurea or with insulin, or conventional policy with diet. Over 10 years, average haemoglobin A1c (HbA$_{1c}$) was 7.0% in the intensive group compared with 7.9% in the conventional group. Compared with the conventional group, the risk in the intensive group was 12% lower (95% Confidence Interval [CI] 1–21, p=0.029) for any diabetes-related endpoint; 10% lower (95% CI 11–27, p=0.34) for any diabetes-related death, and 6% lower (95% CI 10–20, p=0.44) for all cause mortality. Most of the risk reduction in the any diabetes-related aggregate endpoint was due to a 25% risk reduction (95% CI 7–40, p=0.0099) in microvascular endpoints. While the effect of glycaemic control on microvascular complications was readily apparent, the effect on cardiovascular (CV) events was not as evident. The 16% reduction in the risk of myocardial infarction recorded during the trial was only close to statistical significance (P=0.052).

The issue was not solved by the results of the Kumamoto study. In this trial, Japanese patients on intensive insulin treatment achieved much better glycaemic control (HbA$_{1c}$ 7.1% vs. 9.45%) than those on conventional insulin therapy. In the former, cumulative percentages of the development and the progression in retinopathy, nephropathy and neuropathy were significantly lower. Based on these results the investigators suggested that treatment should aim at HbA$_{1c}$ <6.5%, fasting blood glucose <6.1 mmol/l, and 2-h post-prandial blood glucose concentration <10 mmol/l as glycaemic thresholds to prevent the onset and the progression of diabetic microangiopathy. After 8-year follow-up, the number of cardiovascular events was ≈50% lower in the intensive group. Unfortunately, the absolute number of events was too small to allow formal statistical analysis so that no final conclusion could be drawn.

3.2.2 **The PROactive study**

The Kumamoto study was carried out in Japanese patients who have features (they are leaner, more insulin deficient, with less dyslipidemia . . .) slightly different from the common Caucasian T2DM patient. Moreover, that was a small trial (n=110) with no power to establish the impact of glycaemic control on CV events. The PROactive trial, in contrast, enrolled 5,238 T2DM patients who had evidence of macrovascular disease. Patients were assigned to oral pioglitazone or matching placebo, to be taken in addition to their glucose-lowering drugs and other medications. During the 34.5 month average time of observation there was no significant reduction in the CV risk in patients in the pioglitazone group (Hazard Ratio [HR] 0.90, 95% CI 0.80–1.02, p=0.095) although statistical significance was achieved for pre-defined secondary endpoint, a composite of all-cause mortality, non-fatal myocardial infarction, and stroke (HR 0.84, 95% CI 0.72–0.98, p=0.027). In summary, the PROactive could not prove, beyond any doubt, that intensive glycaemic control provides a solid benefit in preventing or reducing CV risk in T2DM patients.

3.2.3 **The mega-trials**

This uncertainty has triggered the initiation of three large trials that recruited a total of 23,000 T2DM patients. In the *Action in Diabetes and Vascular Disease: Preterax and Diamicron Modified Release Controlled Evaluation* (ADVANCE) study, a lower mean HbA_{1c} level was achieved in the intensive-control group than in the standard-control group (6.6 *vs.* 7.3%). Intensive control reduced the incidence of combined major macro- and micro-vascular events (HR 0.90, 95% CI 0.82–0.98; p=0.01), as well as that of major microvascular events (HR 0.86, 95% CI, 0.77–0.97; p=0.01). In contrast, there was no significant effect of glucose control on major macro-vascular events, death from cardiovascular causes, or death from any cause. In the *Veteran Administration Diabetes Trial* (VADT), median HbA_{1c} levels were 8.4% in the standard-therapy group and 6.9% in the intensive-therapy group. There was no significant difference between the two groups in the rate of CV events or in the rate of death from any cause (HR 1.07, 95% CI 0.81–1.42; p=0.62). No differences between the two groups were observed for microvascular complications as well, with the exception of reduced progression diabetic nephropathy. Finally, the *Action to Control Cardiovascular Risk in Diabetes* (ACCORD) study was prematurely interrupted because of a 22% excess risk mortality (95% CI 1.01–1.46) in the intensively treated group. A more recent post-hoc analysis concluded that intensive therapy delayed the onset of albuminuria and some measures of eye complications and neuropathy. The investigators concluded that intensive glycaemic control could provide some microvascular benefits and that this advantage must be weighed against the increase in total and CV-related mortality, increased weight gain, and risk for severe hypoglycaemia.

3.3 Interpreting trials' results

3.3.1 Is it worth to pursue tight glycaemic control?

Some of the features of the above mentioned trials should be critically analysed before a final conclusion is drawn. A careful look at the diabetic population included in the ACCORD, ADVANCE, and VADT trials shows that patients had high CV risk and no less than 35% of them had a previous CV event. It is not surprising that much care was paid in reducing LDL-cholesterol (~2.3 mmol/l) and blood pressure (~120/70 mmHg), in using anti-platelet therapy (62–93% of the patients) and in reducing smoking (8–17%). This multifactorial intervention has been already shown to be effective and it accounts for a very low incidence of CV events in those trials (~2.2% per year). Because of that the room left for a beneficial effect of tight glycaemic control becomes quite narrow requiring either much larger and/or longer studies. However, when patients without a prior CV event were evaluated, tight glycaemic control was associated with a significant reduction of the HR for primary CV outcomes. A similar reduction was apparent when patients with HbA_{1c} ≤8.0% at entry were compared with those with values ≥8.0%. One may assume that the lack of prior CV events or microvascular complications and a lower baseline HbA_{1c} may also reflect a shorter duration of the disease (Figure 3.1). Duration of diabetes may be key in interpreting the results of the recent trials. In these studies strict glycaemic control was achieved, but this happened after years of uncontrolled diabetes. It is readily apparent that this time course is far from the ideal, i.e. the early achievement and maintenance of near-normal glycaemia from the time of diagnosis. The difference between the ideal and the actual time course of glycaemic control represents a time period (Figure 3.2) that 1. leads to the development of diabetic complications and 2. generate a 'bad glycaemic legacy'. This is specular to the 'legacy effect' proposed by the post-trial results of the UKPDS: intensive treatment implemented at the time of the diagnosis results in a sustained reduction in the risk of micro-as well as macrovascular complications. In the 10 year post-trial follow-up, patients originally randomized to receive intensive treatment, not only still showed significant reductions in the rates of diabetes-related endpoints and microvascular complications, but were also at reduced risk of myocardial infarction (relative risk (RR) reduction 15%; $p=0.0014$) and all-cause mortality (RR reduction 13%; $p=0.007$). The relationship between diabetes duration before initiating intensive treatment and

	UKPDS (n=3867)	ADVANCE (n=11,140)	ACCORD (n=10,251)	VADT (n=1791)
Duration of diabetes (years)	0	8	10	11.5
Mean baseline HbA_{1c} (%)	7.1	7.5	8.3	9.4
Mean baseline FPG (mmol/L)	8.0	8.5	9.7	11.4
Mean age (years)	53	66	62	60
Micro	↓	↓	=↓	=
Macro	↓	=	↑	=

Fig 3.1 Compared with the pivotal UKPDS study, which enrolled newly diagnosed patients, recent trials have enrolled higher-risk patient populations characterized by a longer duration of disease, older age and more severe hyperglycaemia (HbA_{1c}) at baseline. Data from The ADVANCE Collaborative Group (2008), VADT Investigators (2008), and The ACCORD Study Group (2008).

outcomes is apparent from Figure 3.1: the longer the duration, the less the effect of tight glycaemic control on diabetic complication. This view should lead to a true change in the treatment strategy of T2DM, that is implementation of appropriate treatment at the time of diagnosis and reduction of treatment associated-risk in those with long-standing disease. Early intervention is safer and more effective because the probability of diabetic complications at diagnosis is low. The 'metabolic legacy' is short in duration and, hence, easier to be modified. In these patients, therefore, targeting normoglycaemia is not just feasible but mandatory. In all cases, an uncompromised

45

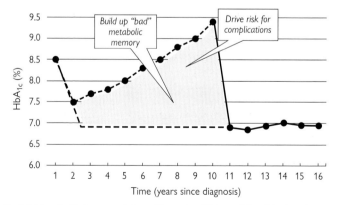

Fig 3.2 Hypothetical representation of the natural history of the diabetic patients recruited in the VADT. The upper dotted line represents the time course of HbA_{1c} estimated on the basis of the average glucose profile described by the UKPDS. The lower dotted line represents the ideal time course of glycaemic control. The solid line represents the time course of HbA_{1c} in the VADT. With kind permission from Springer Science+Business Media: *Diabetologia*, Megatrials in type 2 diabetes. From excitement to frustration?, **52**, 2009, 1219–1226, S. Del Prato, figure 2/.

therapeutic insistence should be adopted, including the treatment of all CV risk factors.

Early intervention is safer and more effective because the probability of diabetes complications at diagnosis is low. This is supported by the ORIGIN trial using the basal insulin analogue, insulin glargine (Lantus®) when its early use was associated with no evidence for increased cardiovascular risk or cancer but there was generally sustained glycaemic control and extremely low rates of hypoglycaemia.

3.3.2 **Is tight glycaemic potentially dangerous?**

In the ACCORD trial tight glycaemic control was associated with an excess of 52 deaths raising the suspicion that aggressive glycaemic control could bring some unwanted risk. This view seemed to be supported by recent data by Currie and co-workers. They assessed survival according to HbA_{1c} in 27,965 T2DM patients whose treatment was intensified from oral monotherapy to combination therapy with oral blood-glucose-lowering agents, and 20,005 patients who changed to treatment regimens that included insulin. The analysis confirmed the association between high HbA_{1c} values and all-cause mortality and CV events, but also highlighted a similar association for low HbA_{1c} values (<7.5%). However, some caution should be used in interpreting these results. First of all, this is not an intervention randomized placebo-controlled study, rather a retrospective analysis with all the caveats this may carry. Moreover, a closer look at the study cohorts reveals some interesting finding. For instance, in patients switched from monotherapy to combined anti-hyperglycaemic therapy there was an inverse relationship between age and HbA_{1c}: the lower the HbA_{1c}, the older the patients. Finally, the percentage of people with increased serum creatinine levels was higher in those with lower HbA_{1c} values suggesting a more severe impairment of the kidney function. Interestingly, both age and glomerular filtration rate are independent predictors of CV mortality. The reason for those associations is not readily apparent, but one may argue that these are the most vulnerable patients in whom aggressive anti-hyperglycaemic treatment may actually expose them to unwanted risk.

The concept of the vulnerable T2DM patient has received support in a recent post-hoc analysis of the ACCORD trial showing that the relationships between average HbA_{1c} and mortality differed between treatment strategies. With the intensive strategy, the risk of death increased continuously from 6.0 to 9.0% average HbA_{1c}, whereas the curve for the standard strategy was distinctly nonlinear. The excess risk associated with intensive glycaemic treatment occurred among those participants whose average HbA_{1c}, contrary to the intent of the strategy, was >7%. In these patients treatment may have become heroic and riskier. Of interest, in the ACCORD study the risk of hypoglycaemia was directly related with HbA_{1c} levels: the less the response on glycaemic control, the

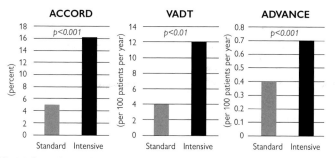

Fig 3.3 Rate of severe hypoglycemia in the ACCORD, VADT and ADVANCE. In the latter the absolute rate was much lower as compared to ACCORD and VADT. However, also in AVANCE the rate of hypoglycaemia was significantly higher in intensively treated patients. Data from The ADVANCE Collaborative Group (2008), VADT Investigators (2008), and The ACCORD Study Group (2008).

more aggressive the treatment, and therefore, the greater the risk of hypoglycaemia. This risk may become dramatic in the elderly, in those with co-morbidities (and multiple pharmacologic treatments), and impaired kidney function.

3.3.3 Is hypoglycaemia responsible for the excess of CV events during intensive therapy?

Hypoglycaemia has been claimed to be a potential CV event trigger in T2DM. Hypoglycaemia was more prevalent in the intensively treated patients in the recent trials (Figure 3.3). Although not completely proven in these trials, hypoglycaemia may be a trigger factor of CV events in vulnerable patients. Low blood glucose levels can activate the nervous autonomic system with 10 to 50 fold increased secretion of catecholamines, cause impaired flexibility in substrate shift in the diabetic myocardium, QTc prolongation and cardiac rate/rhythm disturbances, and excessive glucose fluctuations with marked activation of oxidative stress. A most recent analysis of the ACCORD data has clearly indicated that the mortality rate is higher in those with hypoglycaemia regardless of intensity of treatment. Yet, it was readily apparent that in those with hypoglycaemia, the mortality rate was lower in people with tight as opposed to those with a looser glycaemic control. Similar results have been found in the ADVANCE study. During follow-up, severe hypoglycaemia was associated with a significant increase in the adjusted risks of major macrovascular and microvascular events as well as CV death or from any cause ($p<0.001$ for all comparisons). However, among patients reporting severe hypoglycaemia, annual death rates were lower in the group receiving intensive treatment than in the group receiving standard treatment (3.6 vs. 5.1%). Of interest, hypoglycaemia was also associated to a range of nonvascular outcomes, including respiratory, digestive, and skin conditions ($p<0.01$ for all comparisons). In summary, although it is possible that severe hypoglycaemia may contribute to adverse outcomes, it is also likely that it may be a marker of more vulnerable subjects. On a practical ground, reducing the risk of hypoglycaemia appears to be of importance, and a way to reduce it is to identify patients at increased risk, i.e. the most vulnerable ones. Once again, it is the ACCORD study that gives indication that may help to identify those subjects, since the risk of hypoglycaemia was greater in patients with impaired renal function, with longer duration of diabetes, and in the older ones.

3.3.4 **How much does body weight gain contribute to the risk of intensive therapy?**

Intensive glycaemic control is often associated with an increase in body weight. In the ACCORD more than 25% of the intensively treated patients gained 10 kg over the study period, while in the VADT the average weight gain was >8 kg. To which extent this increase in body weight may have affected the CV outcome remains a matter of debate. In the UKPDS, in the face of an average 5 kg body weight gain, intensive treatment was associated with significant improvement in the microvascular complications and a non-significant reduction in the risk of myocardial infarction.

The impact of body weight change on CV risk of patients treated with insulin after an acute myocardial infarction has been assessed in a post-hoc analysis of the DIGAMI 2 study. Eight hundred-sixty five patients who survived during 12 months after an acute myocardial infarction without any change in their glucose-lowering therapy were divided into four subgroups according to glucose-lowering treatment: group I, no pharmacological glucose-lowering treatment; group II, oral hypoglycaemic agents; group III, new insulin treatment and group IV, insulin before inclusion continued during the first year of follow up. Patients who started on insulin (group III) experienced an average body weight increase of 2.3 kg during the first year of treatment, whereas weight remained unchanged in groups I, II and IV. The incidence of non-fatal reinfarction was higher in patients started on insulin after the myocardial infarction compared with the other groups. However, when the subjects were grouped in quartiles according to maximal body weight increase, those in the lowest quartile experienced the highest CV mortality. Each kilogram increase in weight reduced the risk for CV death with 6%. The study clearly showed that initiation of insulin treatment after myocardial infarction was associated with a significant increase in weight and incidence of reinfarction. The increase in weight did, however, not explain the increased rate of reinfarction.

Rather than the change in body weight, a greater effect may be attributed to the initial body mass index (BMI). By pooling data from the main intervention trials, a strong association between baseline and CV becomes apparent, suggesting that careful phenotyping of patients may guide in reducing the risk associated with tight glycaemic control.

3.4 **Balancing risk and benefit of glycaemic control**

Glycaemic control is recommended but, as suggested, the expected benefits should be weighed against the potential risk associated with progressive but unsuccessful treatment reinforcement, risk of severe hypoglycaemia, and body weight gain. In other words, the risk-to-benefit ratio must be determined individually for each patient. This approach can only proceed through personalization of the treatment goal and pharmacologic approach.

3.4.1 **Toward a personalized glycaemic control**

In revising the results of the recent trials, the ADA and the American Heart Association (AHA) have released a common statement inviting physicians to identify different HbA$_{1c}$ targets for different diabetic subjects (Figure 3.4). Since the vast majority of the patients enrolled in the intervention trails had long duration of the disease and a large proportion already had long-term complications, they advise that in these patients as well as in those with limited life expectancy and history of severe hypoglycaemia, the target HbA$_{1c}$ should be >7%. On the contrary, in persons with short duration diabetes, long life expectancy, no significant cardiovascular disease and no or modest sign of microvascular complications tighter glycaemic control should be achieved and maintained (HbA$_{1c}$ <7%). In these individuals tight glycaemic control may provide additional microvascular benefit. Moreover, preventing the development of microangiopathic complications can also contribute to reduce CV risk. Both micro- and macrovascular complications share common

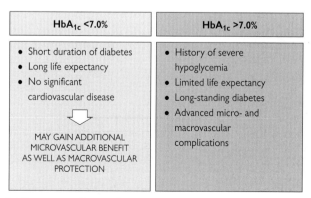

Fig 3.4 Treatment goal personalization according to the American Diabetes Association and the American Heart Association. Reproduced from Skyler JS, Bergenstal R, Bonow RO, et al. (2009).

pathogenetic defects such as oxidative stress. Moreover, microangiopathy is a systemic process involving all body's tissues including the microvasculature of the heart. Such an involvement can contribute to worsen the outcome of atherogenic processes at the level of the coronary arteries and cumulate on the effect of traditional CV risk factors. In keeping with this hypothesis diabetic retinopathy, as well as other microvascular complications, have been shown to be a strong predictor of CV events.

3.4.2 Beyond traditional treatment algorithms. The *ABCD* of glycaemia management

Personalizing treatment may sound rational but it is not necessary a simple exercise. A number of guidelines are available, but, by their nature, they tend to restrict rather than engage therapeutic options. Yet if we pay little attention to what we have so far discussed some elements can be identified that may help guiding treatment selection. These elements include age (A), Body weight (B), Complications (C), and Duration of diabetes (D). Age can be arbitrarily categorized as young (below 40), middle age, and elderly (<70): individualized glycaemic target and the speed of attainment of those targets can be selected based on this simple categorization (Figure 3.5). Body weight may also help in guiding initial pharmacologic intervention as body weight may reflect pronounced insulin resistance and differential CV risk profile. Complications must be evaluated not only in term of increased CV and hypoglycaemia risk but also in term of treatment selection. Duration is likely to be directly associated with the presence of co-morbidities and complications: this will require accurate treatment tuning to reduce the

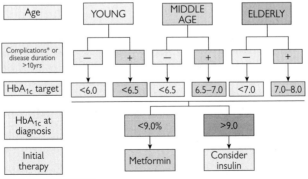

*Micro- and macrovascular complications

Fig 3.5 The HbA$_{1c}$ and ABCD strategy for recently diagnosed patients with T2DM. Adapted from Pozzilli P, Leslie RD, Chan J *et al.* (2010).

risk of severe hypoglycaemia. In other words, drug selection and the HbA$_{1c}$ target should reflect the clinical status of each particular individual. Therefore, for patients prone to hypoglycaemia, careful evaluation of pharmacological treatment is recommended. In summary, age, body weight, concomitant complications and diabetes duration can direct the drug selection by the clinician. A summary for such a decision flow chart at diagnosis is illustrated in Figure 3.5 where indications for considering use of insulin is also given in the case of very poor glycaemic control.

We still remain convinced that the best interpretation of the recent intervention trial has been provided by one of the VADT principal investigator when in the press conference that followed the release of the results commented: 'If you go into a population that already has multiple risk factors—or prior cardiovascular disease—and longstanding poor glucose control, you cannot expect benefits from glucose control in the short term. You can't expect miracles'. Therefore the main lesson of these trials is the need for early and effective intervention. It is worth keeping in mind that no form of mild diabetes exists, and no excuse exists to postpone such an appropriate and effective treatment.

References

Aas AM, Ohrvik J, Malmberg K, Rydén L, Birkeland KI (2009) DIGAMI 2 Investigators. Insulin-induced weight gain and cardiovascular events in patients with type 2 diabetes. A report from the DIGAMI 2 study. *Diabetes Obes Metab* **11**: 323–9.

ACCORD Study Group (2008) Effects of intensive glucose lowering in type 2 diabetes. *N Engl J Med* **358**: 2545–59.

ADVANCE Collaborative Group (2008) Intensive blood glucose control and vascular outcomes in patients with type 2 diabetes. *N Engl J Med* **24**: 739–43.

Bonds DE, Miller ME, Bergenstal RM, *et al.* (2010) The association between symptomatic, severe hypoglycaemia and mortality in type 2 diabetes: retrospective epidemiological analysis of the ACCORD study. *BMJ* **340**: b4909.

Currie CJ, Peters JR, Tynan A, *et al* (2010) Survival as a function of HbA(1c) in people with type 2 diabetes: a retrospective cohort study. *Lancet* **375**: 481–9.

Del Prato S (2009) Megatrials in type 2 diabetes. From excitement to frustration? *Diabetologia* **52**: 1219–26.

Del Prato S, LaSalle J, Matthaei S, Bailey CJ (2010) Global Partnership for Effective Diabetes Management. Tailoring treatment to the individual in type 2 diabetes practical guidance from the Global Partnership for Effective Diabetes Management. *Int J Clin Pract* **64**: 295–304.

Dormandy JA, Charbonnel B, Eckland DJ (2005) Secondary prevention of macrovascular events in patients with type 2 diabetes in the PROactive Study (PROspective pioglitAzone Clinical Trial In macroVascular Events): a randomised controlled trial. *Lancet* **366**: 1279–89.

Duckworth W, Abraira C, Moritz T, *et al.* (2008) VADT Investigators. Glucose control and vascular complications in veterans with type 2 diabetes. *N Engl J Med* **358**: 2560–72.

Holman RR, Paul SK, Bethel MA, *et al.* (2008) 10-year follow-up of intensive glucose control in type 2 diabetes. *N Engl J Med* **359**: 1577–89.

Ismail-Beigi F, Craven T, Banerji MA, *et al.* (2001) Effect of intensive treatment of hyperglycaemia on microvascular outcomes in type 2 diabetes: an analysis of the ACCORD randomised trial. *Lancet* **376**: 419–30.

Juutilainen A, Lehto S, Rönnemaa T, Pyörälä K, Laakso M (2007) Retinopathy predicts cardiovascular mortality in type 2 diabetic men and women. *Diabetes Care* **30**: 292–9.

Mannucci E, Monami M, Lamanna C, Gori F, Marchionni N (2009) Prevention of cardiovascular disease through glycemic control in type 2 diabetes: a meta-analysis of randomized clinical trials. *Nutr Metab Cardiovasc Dis* **19**: 604–12.

Miller ME, Bonds DE, Gerstein HC, *et al.* (2010) ACCORD Investigators. The effects of baseline characteristics, glycaemia treatment approach, and glycated haemoglobin concentration on the risk of severe hypoglycaemia: post hoc epidemiological analysis of the ACCORD study. *BMJ* **340**: b5444.

Ohkubo Y, Kishikawa H, Araki E, *et al.* (1995) Intensive insulin therapy prevents the progression of diabetic microvascular complications in Japanese patients with non-insulin-dependent diabetes mellitus: a randomized prospective 6-year study. *Diabetes Res Clin Prac* **28**: 103–17.

Origin Trial Investigators (2012) Basal insulin and cardiovascular and other outcomes in dysglycemia. *New England Journal of Medicine* **367**: 319–28.

Origin Trial Investigators (2008) Rationale, design, and baseline characteristics for a large international trial of cardiovascular disease prevention in people with dysglycemia: The ORIGIN Trial (Outcome Reduction with an Initial Glargine Intervention). *American Heart Journal* **155**: 26–32.

Pozzilli P, Leslie RD, Chan J, De Fronzo R, Monnier L, Raz I, Del Prato S (2010) The A1C and ABCD of glycaemia management in type 2 diabetes: a physician's personalized approach. *Diabetes Metab Res Rev* **26**: 239–44.

Riddle MC, Ambrosius WT, Brillon DJ, *et al.* (2010) Action to Control Cardiovascular Risk in Diabetes Investigators Epidemiologic relationships between A1C and all-cause mortality during a median 3.4-year follow-up of glycemic treatment in the ACCORD trial. *Diabetes Care* **33**: 983–90.

Shichiri M, Kishikawa H, Ohkubo Y, Wake N (2000) Long-term results of the Kumamoto Study on optimal diabetes control in type 2 diabetic patients. *Diabetes Care* **23**: B21–B29.

Skyler JS, Bergenstal R, Bonow RO, *et al.* (2009) Intensive glycemic control and the prevention of cardiovascular events: implications of the ACCORD, ADVANCE, and VA Diabetes Trials: a position statement of the American

Diabetes Association and a Scientific Statement of the American College of Cardiology Foundation and the American Heart Association. *J Am Coll Cardiol.* **53**: 298–304.

UK Prospective Diabetes Study (UKPDS) Group (1988) Intensive blood-glucose control with sulphonylureas or insulin compared with conventional treatment and risk of complications in patients with type 2 diabetes (UKPDS 33). *Lancet* **352**: 837–53.

Zoungas S, Patel A, Chalmers J, *et al.* (2010) ADVANCE Collaborative Group. Severe hypoglycemia and risks of vascular events and death. *N Engl J Med* **363**: 1410–18.

Chapter 4

Pharmacotherapy in type 2 diabetes: clinical evidence

Gayatri Sreemantula, Santosh Shankarnarayan, and Jiten P Vora

Key points

- Patients with type 2 diabetes demonstrate increased cardiovascular risk; this risk is significantly reduced by improved glycaemic control
- Recent trials have demonstrated that both low and high mean HbA_{1c} values are associated with increased all-cause mortality and cardiac events
- UKPDS and further Cochrane analysis showed that metformin improves glycaemia, is weight neutral and possesses positive cardiovascular profile. Lactic acidosis, in one systematic analysis, is proved to be extremely rare and prevalence may be similar to placebo in low risk groups
- Thiazolidinediones are efficacious, combine well with other agents for diabetes and show good durability, They are associated with weight gain, increase risk of (non-fatal) heart failure and increase risk of small bone fracture in women. Rosiglitazone (but not pioglitazone) has been associated with increased risk of myocardial infarction and the European Medicines Agency has recently recommended suspension of all authorization of its use
- Sulfonylureas are efficacious, with rapid onset of action and combine well with other agents for diabetes in the European Union diabetes. They are associated with weight gain and increased risk of hypoglycaemia

- Initial addition of basal insulin to oral therapy followed by subsequent intensification to a basal-prandial regimen would be the ideal insulin treatment strategy
- Current evidence is suggestive of a potential association between use of analogue insulins and increased cancer incidence and would warrant further investigations.

4.1 Introduction

The prevalence of diabetes continues to increase worldwide. Currently, about 5% (285 million) of the global population is affected, approximately 85% of whom have type 2 diabetes. Since 1996 in the UK alone, the number of people diagnosed with diabetes has increased from 1.4 million to 2.65 million. It has been estimated that by 2025 over 4 million people will have diabetes. The Framingham heart study suggested that patients with diabetes carried increased cardiovascular risk, which is comparable to those without diabetes but with known cardiovascular disease (Figure 4.1). Similarly people with type 2 diabetes have a two-fold increased risk of stroke within the first 5 years of diagnosis compared with the general population.

The benefits of improved glycaemic control have been unequivocally demonstrated in both types 1 and 2 diabetes. The Diabetes Control and Complications Trial (DCCT) demonstrated that intensive therapy to improve glycaemic control in patients with type 1 diabetes mellitus reduces the risk of microvascular disease, and may also reduce the risk of macrovascular disease (The Diabetes Control and Complications Trial Research Group, 1993); intensive therapy also reduced the adjusted mean risk for the development

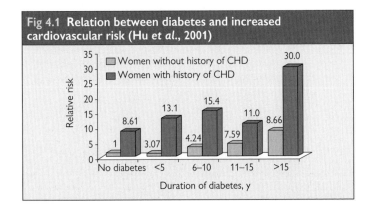

Fig 4.1 **Relation between diabetes and increased cardiovascular risk (Hu et al., 2001)**

of retinopathy by 76% (95% CI 62–85%), slowed the progression of retinopathy by 54% (95% CI 39–66%), reduced the development of proliferative or severe non-proliferative retinopathy by 47% (95% CI 14–67%) and reduced the occurrence of microalbuminuria (urinary albumin excretion of 40 mg per 24 hours) by 39% (95% CI 21–52%), that of albuminuria (urinary albumin excretion of 300 mg per 24 hours) by 54% (95% CI 19–74%) and that of clinical neuropathy by 60% (95% CI 38–74%). Similarly, in type 2 diabetes, The United Kingdom Prospective Diabetes Study (UKPDS) demonstrated that intensive glycaemic control significantly reduces both micro- and macro-vascular complications (Figure 4.2); epidemiological extrapolation suggested that for every 1% reduction in HbA_{1c} there would be reduction in risk of 21% for any end point related to diabetes (95% CI 17–24%, $p<0.0001$), 21% for deaths related to diabetes (15–27%, $p<0.0001$), 14% for myocardial infarction (8–21%, $p<0.0001$) and 37% for microvascular complications (33–41%, $p<0.0001$) (Stratton *et al.*, 2000) (Table 4.1).

The UKPDS also assisted in clarifying the pathophysiology of type 2 diabetes. Key abnormalities in the development of type 2 diabetes are insulin resistance and beta-cell dysfunction (defects of

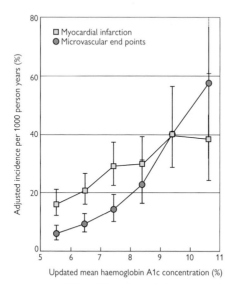

Fig 4.2 Incidence rates and 95% confidence intervals for myocardial infarction and microvascular complications by category of updated mean haemoglobin A1c concentration, adjusted for age, sex, and ethnic group, expressed for white men aged 50–54 years at diagnosis and with mean duration of diabetes of 10 years. Reproduced from *British Medical Journal*, Irene M Stratton, Amanda I Adler, H Andrew W Neil, David R Matthews, Susan E Manley, Carole A Cull, David Hadden, Robert C Turner, Rury R Holman, **321**: 405–412, copyright 2000 with permission from BMJ Publishing Group Ltd.

Table 4.1 Observational analysis of relation between glycaemic exposure and complications of diabetes as estimated by decrease in risk for 1% reduction in haemoglobin A1c (HbA$_{1c}$) concentration, measured at baseline and as updated mean, controlled for age at diagnosis of diabetes, sex, ethnic group, smoking, albuminuria, systolic blood pressure, high- and low-density lipoprotein cholestrol, and triglycerides (n = 3642) compared with results of clinical trial of intensive versus conventional glucose control policy (n = 3867)

| | Observational analysis | | | | Clinical trial of intensive versus conventional policy[1] | | |
| | Baseline HbA$_{1c}$ | | Updated mean HbA$_{1c}$ | | | | |
	No of events	Decrease in risk (%)/1% reduction (95% CI)	p value	Decrease in risk (%)/1% reduction (95% CI)	p value	No of events	Decrease in risk (%) seen for 0.9% difference in HbA$_{1c}$ (95% CI)	p value
Aggregate and points								
Any end point related to diabetes	1255	11 (8 to 13)	<0.0001	21 (17 to 24)	<0.0001	1401	12 (1 to 21)	0.029
Deaths related to diabetes	346	9 (3 to 14)	0.0018	21 (15 to 27)	<0.0001	414	10 (−11 to 27)	0.34
All cause mortality	597	6 (2 to 10)	0.0081	14 (9 to 19)	<0.0001	702	6 (−10 to 20)	0.44
All cause mortality	597	6 (2 to 10)	0.0081	14 (9 to 19)	<0.0001	702	6 (10 to 20)	0.44

Myocardial infarction	496	5 (0 to 9)	0.067	14 (8 to 21)	<0.0001	573	16 (0 to 29)	0.052
Stroke	162	−4 (−14 to 6)	0.44	12 (1 to 21)	0.035	203	−11 (−49 to 19)	0.52
Peripheral vascular disease*	41	28 (18 to 37)	<0.0001	43 (31 to 53)	<0.0001	47	35 (18 to 64)	0.15
Microvascular disease	323	23 (20 to 27)	<0.0001	37 (33 to 41)	<0.0001	346	25 (7 to 40)	0.0099
Single end points							
Heart failure	104	0 (−12 to 11)	0.99	16 (3 to 26)	0.016	116	9 (−35 to 39)	0.63
Cataract extraction	195	9 (2 to 16)	0.013	19 (11 to 26)	<0.0001	229	24 (0 to 42)	0.046

*Lower extremity amputation or fatal peripheral vascular disease. Reproduced from *British Medical Journal*, Irene M Stratton, Amanda I Adler, H Andrew W Neil, David R Matthews, Susan E Manley, Carole A Cull, David Hadden, Robert C Turner, Rury R Holman, **321**: 405–412, copyright 2000 with permission from BMJ Publishing Group Ltd.

insulin secretion). Considerable debate continues as to whether insulin resistance is the primary culprit followed by defects in insulin secretion. It is for this reason that many investigators have focused on the stage of impaired glucose tolerance that is prior to the development of frank diabetes. However, for type 2 diabetes the key issue remains that beta-cell dysfunction, and consequent defective insulin secretion, exacerbate the effects of insulin resistance (insulin action). The primary glucose-lowering effects of insulin are suppression of hepatic glucose output (by stimulating glycogen synthesis, reducing both glycogenolysis and gluconeogenesis) and stimulation of glucose uptake and oxidation predominantly by skeletal muscle and adipose tissue. Hepatic glucose production is a major determinant of fasting plasma glucose levels. In type 2 diabetes there is increased hepatic glucose production due to insulin resistance, resulting in inadequate suppression of gluconeogenesis. Consequently, the presence of fasting hyperinsulinaemia in the presence of a normal or elevated plasma glucose level indicates insulin resistance. Insulin action throughout the body may be reduced because of a combination of pre-receptor, receptor or post-receptor defects. Whilst glucose uptake requires higher levels of insulin than those for suppression of hepatic glucose output, such defects result in reduced glucose disposal. Indeed, one of the key effects of insulin is to induce translocation of the GLUT4 glucose transporter in skeletal muscle, alteration of which results in reduced glucose uptake.

In the presence of insulin resistance, compensatory increase in insulin secretion initially maintains glucose levels within the normal range. However, protracted hyperglycaemia is not associated with continual increases in insulin secretion and eventually insulin secretion becomes defective and hyperglycaemia escalates. Early abnormalities of insulin secretion, including prior to the development of frank diabetes, are often seen in first-degree relatives of patients with diabetes, include loss of the normal pulsatility and impairment of the first phase of insulin secretion and defective beta-cell processing of proinsulin, resulting in increased secretion of proinsulin-like molecules. The UKPDS also clearly demonstrated that one of the characteristic features of type 2 diabetes is the progressive decline in pancreatic beta-cell function resulting in most patients invariably requiring pharmacological treatment and eventually insulin therapy. Additionally, it appears that there are currently no therapies that modify the individual rates of decline of beta-cell function. Hence, whilst diet, lifestyle intervention, self management and structured patient education remain the cornerstones of diabetes care, better understanding of pharmaco-therapeutic agents in type 2 diabetes is pivotal in the clinical care of people with type 2 diabetes.

In addition to traditional oral anti-diabetes agents (OADs) (biguanides and sulfonylureas), thiazolidinediones, prandial glucose regulators and alpha-glucosidase inhibitors are also used either alone or as combination therapy. In spite of the wide range of options for multiple OHAs, optimal glycaemic control is often not achieved and the majority of patients eventually need insulin. Efforts to maintain long-term stable glycaemic control is frequently hampered by weight gain associated with most anti-diabetes medications, increasing the level of insulin resistance and progressive pancreatic beta-cell dysfunction. Thus, there have been continuous efforts to achieve an ideal anti-diabetes therapy/regime that provides adequate and stable glycaemic control, maintains weight, treats the pre-existent insulin resistance, preserves beta-cell function, reduces cardiovascular risk and demonstrates appropriate levels of safety. The recent introduction of newer anti-diabetes agents (incretin-based therapies and soon SGLT2 inhibitors) have widened the therapeutic options available to achieve optimal glycaemic control. Further, the incretin-based therapies show promise because of weight reduction or a weight-neutral effect but long-term safety and cardiovascular risk reduction data are awaited.

4.2 Biguanides

Metformin is the only biguanide widely used in routine clinical management of diabetes and is the treatment of choice for overweight people with type 2 diabetes in whom it is weight neutral (Hermann et al., 1994) or produces modest weight loss in contrast to sulfonylureas, thiazolidinediones or insulin, which may produce weight gain. Further advantages include a low risk of hypoglycaemia and a small beneficial effect on lipid profile (Wu et al., 1990). However, as with other OADs, loss of glycaemic control is commonly also observed over time. A retrospective analysis demonstrated that patients commenced on metformin tend to achieve maximum reduction in HbA_{1c} after 6 months. For patients taking metformin and thiazolidinedione, this reduction was maintained at 9 months. However, for patients taking a sulfonylurea, a trend for HbA_{1c} values to increase was evident by 9 months. The rate of secondary failure for patients taking metformin (35.5%) was lower than the rate for those taking a sulfonylurea (40.7%, $p = 0.011$) and similar to the rate for patients taking a thiazolidinedione (30.6%) (Wu et al., 1990).

In one observational study, (Brown et al., 2004) metformin failure occurred more rapidly in clinical practice than in clinical trials (42% vs. 35.5%, mean failure rate 17% per year). However, patients who initiated metformin within 3 months of diabetes diagnosis and patients who initiated metformin while HbA_{1c} was <7% failed at a much lower adjusted rate of 12.2% (10.5–14.4%) per year, and 12.3% per year respectively.

A secondary analysis of the UKPDS suggested reduced cardiovascular risk with metformin compared to conventional therapy in a small number of patients; metformin therapy was associated with significant relative risk reductions of 32% for any diabetes-related end point, 42% for diabetes-related death and 36% for all-cause mortality (Riedel et al., 2007). Likewise, metformin also demonstrated superiority for any diabetes-related end points and all-cause mortality, compared to intensive therapy with sulfonylurea or insulin ($p = 0.003$). In addition, a Cochrane review on metformin monotherapy reported greater benefit in obese patients allocated to intensive blood glucose control with metformin compared with chlorpropamide, glibenclamide or insulin for any diabetes-related outcomes ($p = 0.009$) and for all-cause mortality ($p = 0.03$). Obese participants assigned to intensive blood glucose control with metformin showed a greater benefit than overweight patients on conventional treatment for any diabetes related outcomes ($p = 0.004$), diabetes-related death ($p = 0.03$), all-cause mortality ($p = 0.01$) and myocardial infarction ($p = 0.02$) (Saenz et al., 2007) (Figure 4.3). However more recently a double-blind randomized controlled trial, A Diabetes Outcome Progression Trial (ADOPT), reported that the sulfonylurea (glibenclamide (glyburide)) was associated with a lower risk of cardiovascular events (including congestive heart failure) than was rosiglitazone and metformin ($p<0.05$), whilst the latter two demonstrated similar risk (Kahn et al., 2007).

Lactic acidosis is probably the most notorious and potentially serious side effect of metformin though one large systematic review suggested that lactic acidosis is extremely rare and the prevalence may not be any different from placebo (Salpeter et al., 2002). It is recommended however because of the possible increased risk that metformin should not be used in patients with significant renal failure (eGFR <30 ml/min). Traditionally, metformin is considered to be absolutely contraindicated in patients with heart failure. However, a systematic review reported that metformin therapy in patients with heart failure may be associated with lower mortality rates but statistical heterogeneity precluded formal meta-analysis (Evrich et al., 2007).

4.3 **Sulfonylureas**

Worldwide, sulfonylureas are the most commonly used OHAs. They are potent and rapid anti-diabetes agents, reducing fasting glucose (by 20%) and HbA$_{1c}$ (by approximately 1.5%), therefore of particular importance in significant hyperglycaemia where rapid control is required. On the other hand, there is secondary failure, with a rate of 20–40%. In the UKPDS, 53% of newly diagnosed diabetic patients treated with a sulfonylurea required the addition of insulin to

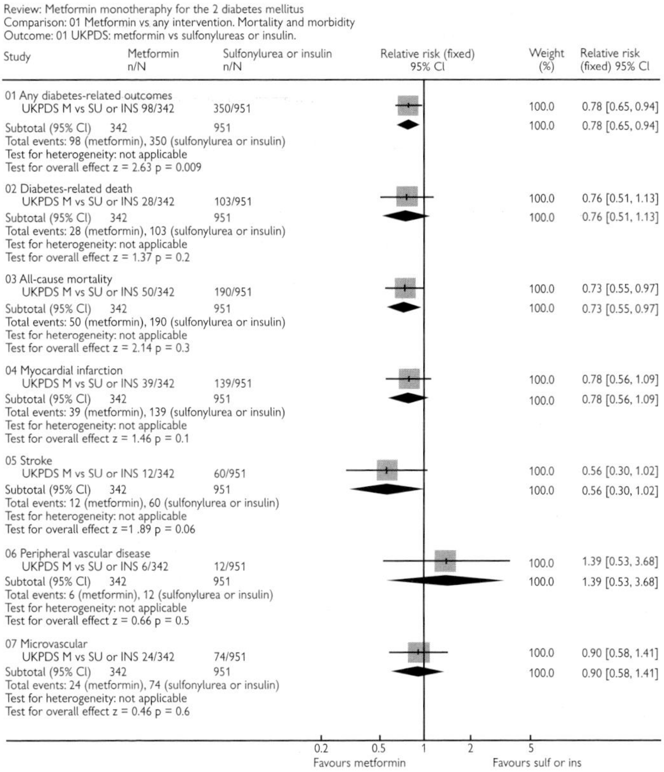

Fig 4.3 Metformin versus sulfonylureas or insulin. Reproduced from A. Saenz *et al.* Metformin monotherapy for type 2 diabetes mellitus.

maintain adequate glycaemic control by 6 years (Wright *et al.*, 2002), a finding that is supported by further controlled trials (Edwards, 2003). This secondary failure rate was also seen when sulfonylureas were used in the combination therapy with metformin (Cook *et al.*, 2005). Hypoglycaemia is the most common and potentially most serious side effect, especially with long-acting sulfonylureas. UKPDS suggested 12.1% per annum hypoglycaemia rate with chlorpropamide and 17.5% with glibenclamide. Shorter acting and newer sulfonylureas cause less hypoglycaemia. However, all sulfonylureas are associated with weight gain, potentially less with the newer agents.

The effect of sulfonylureas on cardiovascular risk is controversial. It has been postulated that sulfonylureas may prevent coronary vasodilatation by action on adenosine triphosphate (ATP)-dependent potassium channels. Increased cardiovascular death was reported with tolbutamide by the University Group Diabetes

Program (UGDP) (Simts and Thien, 1995) over 20 years ago. The study has been criticized as further studies reported improved survival after myocardial infarction or reduced cardiovascular risk (Paasikivi and Wahlberg, 1971; Sartor, 1980). Concerns raised by the UGDP that sulfonylureas may increase CVD mortality in type 2 diabetes were also not substantiated by the UKPDS or ADVANCE study. A recent retrospective analysis compared individual sulfony-lureas and showed no statistically significant difference in the risk of overall mortality, but did suggest that glimepiride may be the preferred sulfonylurea in patients with underlying coronary artery disease (Pantalone et al., 2010). See also Figure 4.4.

4.4 **Prandial glucose regulators (meglitinides)**

The meglitinides, repaglinide and nateglinide, are short-acting OHAs that stimulate insulin secretion via ATP-dependent potassium chan-nels in a glucose-dependent fashion. Repaglinide licensed to be used as a monotherapy or in combination therapy with metformin. Nateglinide can only be used in combination with metformin. Their clinical efficacy is akin to that of sulfonylureas in both reducing fasting glucose and HbA$_{1c}$ (Wolffenbuttel et al., 1999; Schmitz et al., 2002). There are no long-term studies to evaluate their efficacy or effect on cardiovascular risk. This requires study as they act on potassium channel, similar to the sulfonylureas.

4.5 **Thiazolidinediones (TZDs)**

The TZDs (peroxisome proliferator-activated receptors—PPAR gamma-receptor agonists) were introduced about 10 years ago as a treatment for type 2 diabetes. The heightened insulin sensitivity and ability to improve glycaemic control increased their appeal. They are licensed for use as monotherapy or in combination with metformin, sulfonylurea and DPP4 inhibitors. Their efficacy as monotherapy is similar to metformin, reducing HbA$_{1c}$ by approximately 1–1.5%. Because of their putative effect on pancreatic beta-cell preservation, the effect of TZDs in reducing the progression of impaired fast-ing glycaemia (IFG) or impaired glucose tolerance (IGT) to diabetes has also been examined. The Diabetes REduction Assessment with ramipril and rosiglitazone Medication (DREAM) trial reported that less people with IFG or IGT develop diabetes when treated with rosiglitazone, though this may simply reflect the known glucose low-ering effect of TZDs. The study reported that, in rosiglitazone, the rate of decline of beta-cell function after 6 months and secondary

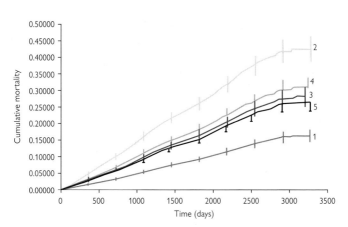

Fig 4.4 Cumulative mortality rates (with standard errors at yearly intervals) in five study cohorts: 1. Metformin monotherapy: patients treated with metformin only. 2. Sulfonylureas monotherapy: patients treated with sulfonylureas only. 3. Combination-1: patients treated with metformin with sulfonylureas added later. 4. Combination-2: patients treated with sulfonylureas with metformin added later. 5. Both: treatment with both sulfonylureas and metformin on the same day.

failure rate after 6 months was lower than those of both sulfonylurea and metformin (Figures 4.5 and 4.6).

The ADOPT study also suggested an increase in distal fractures, which is now felt to reflect PPAR activity on stem cells resulting in increased localized formation of adipose tissue. There is also emerging evidence suggesting that TZDs reduce total body bone mineral

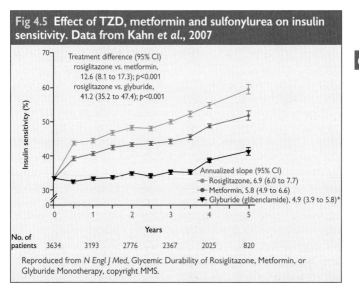

Fig 4.5 Effect of TZD, metformin and sulfonylurea on insulin sensitivity. Data from Kahn et al., 2007

Treatment difference (95% CI)
rosiglitazone vs. metformin,
12.6 (8.1 to 17.3); p<0.001
rosiglitazone vs. glyburide,
41.2 (35.2 to 47.4); p<0.001

Annualized slope (95% CI)
Rosiglitazone, 6.9 (6.0 to 7.7)
Metformin, 5.8 (4.9 to 6.6)
Glyburide (glibenclamide), 4.9 (3.9 to 5.8)*

| No. of patients | 3634 | 3193 | 2776 | 2367 | 2025 | 820 |

Reproduced from *N Engl J Med*, Glycemic Durability of Rosiglitazone, Metformin, or Glyburide Monotherapy, copyright MMS.

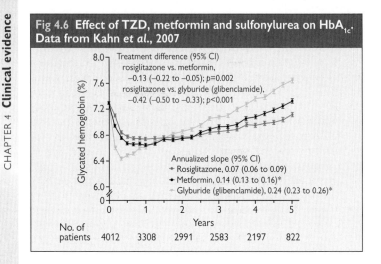

Fig 4.6 **Effect of TZD, metformin and sulfonylurea on HbA₁c. Data from Kahn et al., 2007**

density, the mechanism of which remains to be elucidated (Schwartz et al., 2006; www.fda.gov/MedWatch/index.html).

By nature of their potential anti-inflammatory and anti-thrombotic property (Gervois et al., 2007; Meisner et al., 2006), it was thought that TZDs would not only improve glucose control by targeting insulin resistance, but also reduce cardiovascular events. In a population of 'high-risk' patients with type 2 diabetes (who possessed a history of cardiovascular events), pioglitazone reduced all-cause mortality, fatal and non-fatal myocardial infarction (MI) and stroke by 18% (Dormandy et al., 2005). Indeed, in patients with a previous MI, recurrent fatal/non-fatal MI were reduced by 28% and time to further acute coronary syndrome (ACS) by 37%. In patients with previous stroke, recurrence was reduced by 47%. In contrast, a subsequent integrated clinical trial evaluation of rosiglitazone, undertaken by GlaxoSmithKline, suggested a hazard ratio of 1.31 for myocardial ischaemia.

More recently there have been increasing reports of peripheral oedema and congestive cardiac failure with both drugs (Juurlink, 2010). These effects are thought to be due to the increased salt and water reabsorption at the distal nephron, which is mediated by the activation of PPAR-γ. There have been numerous meta-analyses suggesting either a similar increased hazard ratio or no significant impact of rosiglitazone on major adverse cardiovascular events of myocardial ischemia, stroke and cardiovascular mortality (Nissen and Wolski, 2007; Lincoff et al., 2007). The methodology of such analysis has been repeatedly and frequently criticized, there have been very few events to evaluate, and most importantly most of the studies evaluated in these meta-analyses are of varying duration and not designed to investigate cardiovascular outcomes.

The Rosiglitazone Evaluated for Cardiac Outcomes and Regulation of glycaemia in Diabetes (RECORD) trial, studied long-term effects of the combination of metformin and sulfonylureas versus rosiglitazone and metformin and did not reveal an increase in cardiovascular risk for rosiglitazone (Home et al., 2007). The study was limited by low event rates, which resulted in insufficient statistical power to confirm or refute evidence of an increased risk for ischaemic myocardial events (DeAngelis, 2010; Psaty, 2009; Nissen, 2010).

Pioglitazone has also been subjected to similar meta-analysis, with identical caveats regarding the methodology. However, many of these meta-analyses appear to suggest either no effect or reduced cardiovascular risk associated with treatment with pioglitazone (Dormandy et al., 2005; Lincoff et al., 2007). Both rosiglitazone and pioglitazone have been associated with an increased risk of congestive heart failure. There are several hypotheses to explain this observed difference between the two thiazolidines. Rosiglitazone therapy is associated with a 23% increase in the low-density lipoprotein cholesterol (LDL-C) levels while pioglitazone therapy reduced triglyceride levels and also produced a significantly greater increase in high-density lipoprotein levels. Rosiglitazone activates matrix metalloproteinase 3, an enzyme linked to plaque rupture (Wilson, 2008).

Amidst the controversies around the CV safety of rosiglitazone, it should be noted that there have been no definitive randomized controlled CV outcome trials that can answer this question satisfactorily. A more comprehensive meta-analysis recently published analysed MI and CV mortality for 56 randomized trials involving 35,531 patients showed a significantly increased odds ratio for MI but without evidence of an increase in CV or all-cause mortality. The estimated 28% to 39% increase in the risk for MI observed for rosiglitazone use and the number needed to harm of 52 or 37 (with or without the RECORD trial) represent a significant potential health burden (Nissen, 2010).

Consequently, the Food and Drug Administration in the United States and the European Medicines Agency (EMA) have concluded that the benefits of the TZDs outweigh the risks, although recent labelling now recognizes the possibility of increased cardiovascular risk with rosiglitazone. The FDA has decided that rosiglitazone can remain available, but only under a very stringent restricted-access program. However, the EMA has recommended the suspension of the marketing authorizations for all rosiglitazone-containing antidiabetes medications licensed in the EU.

4.6 **Alpha-glucosidase inhibitors**

Acarbose is the only available alpha-glucosidase inhibitor in the United Kingdom. It reduces the absorption of glucose and control the post-prandial glycaemia, possessing a modest efficacy in reducing HbA_{1c} by 0.77% (Van de Laar et al., 2005) when used as monotherapy or combination therapy with other OHAs. Its effect on lowering fasting glucose is relative smaller than prandial glucose and HbA_{1c} reduction. In the Study to Prevent Non-Insulin Dependent Diabetes Mellitus (STOP-NIDDM) trial, treatment with acarbose led to significant cardiovascular risk reduction (Chiasson et al., 2003) (relative risk reduction 49% and absolute risk reduction 2.5%), which may highlight the importance of post-prandial glycaemia.

4.7 **Insulin**

4.7.1 **When to start insulin in Type 2 diabetes?**

The timing of initiation of insulin therapy has been a subject of much debate. Excellent glycaemic control has been reported when insulin is initiated as first-line therapy when diet and lifestyle measures fail (Li et al., 2004). However, UKPDS does not show any superiority of glycaemic control or quality of life when insulin is used as initial treatment and stated that 'in patients with primary diet failure, it may not be advantageous to proceed directly to insulin therapy. It is reasonable to initiate therapy with oral agents and proceed to insulin if the goal is not achieved.' (UKPDS, 1998) In fact, UKPDS considered the addition of insulin to failing first-line sulfonylurea oral therapy as early treatment and showed that HbA_{1c} could be maintained close to 7% for up to 6 years after diagnosis (Wright et al., 2002). In contrast, most current 'conventional insulin start policy' recommended commencing insulin only when a patient has experienced progressive loss of glycaemic control when using a progressive step-wise introduction of oral agents (mono, dual and triple) by which time the patient has had diabetes for 10–15 years and may potentially have already developed complications such as cardiovascular disease (Nathan, 2002). The introduction of the injectable GLP-1 mimetics (exenatide, liraglutide) now means they are also available as third line therapy. Thus, recently updated consensus guidelines issued by the American Diabetes Association (ADA) and the European Association for the Study of Diabetes (EASD) recommend a step-wise approach to the management of hyperglycaemia in type 2 diabetes by adding in agents when patients fail to achieve adequate glycaemic control (Figure 4.7). Metformin is the generally recommended gold standard first line pharmacotherapy but most importantly the guideline stresses a patient centred approach

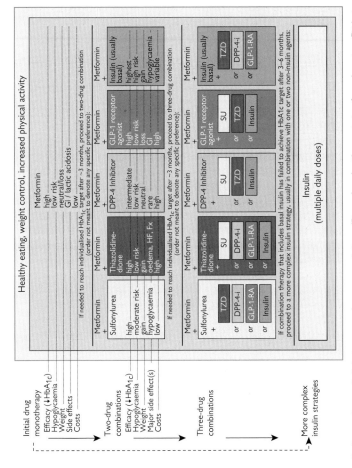
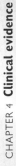
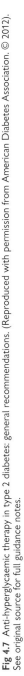

Fig 4.7 Anti-hyperglycaemic therapy in type 2 diabetes: general recommendations. (Reproduced with permission from American Diabetes Association. © 2012). See original source for full guidance notes.

defined as 'providing care which is respectful of and responsive to individual patient preferences, needs, and values, and ensuring that patient values guide all clinical decisions' (this is ref 25 from the document).The guideline recommends that any of the available oral agents can be used second line after metformin as well as injectable GLP-1 agonists depending on individual patient characteristics and preferences. The risks of weight gain are specifically mentioned with sulfonylureas and glitazones and also hypoglycaemia with sulfonylureas versus lack of weight gain and very low risk of hypoglycaemia with DPP-4 inhibitors and GLP-1 agonists. Insulin can be used at any stage including second line especially if the patient is significantly symptomatic and/or the HbA_{1c} is very high. The point is made that insulin remains the most efficacious of all treatments for hyperglycaemia and is commonly started too late after many years of poor glycaemic control ie it should not be a treatment of last resort.

4.7.2 Target HbA_{1c}

HbA_{1c} target should be as close to the non-diabetic range as possible provided that the patient is reasonably free from hypoglycaemia. The retrospective study by Brown et al. (2004) demonstrated that the average patient accumulated nearly 5 HbA_{1c}-years of excess glycaemic burden >8.0% from diagnosis until starting insulin and about 10 HbA_{1c}-years of burden >7.0%. There is an increasing body of evidence indicating that the failed glycaemic control and resultant unacceptable glycaemic burden is associated with an inexorable decline in beta-cell function and both micro- and macrovascular complications.

In a retrospective study of patients with type 2 diabetes, Craig J Currie et al. (2010) demonstrated that a HbA_{1c} of approximately 7.5% (median HbA_{1c} 7.5%, IQR 7.5–7.6%) was associated with lowest all-cause mortality and lowest progression to large vessel disease events. The adjusted hazard ratio (HR) of all-cause mortality in the lowest HbA_{1c} decile (6.4%, 6.1–6.6) was 1.52 (95% CI 1.32–1.76), and in the highest HbA_{1c} decile (median 10.5%, IQR 10.1–11.2%) was 1.79 (95% CI 1.56–2.06). These results showed a U-shaped pattern of risk association, and suggested that an increase or decrease from mean HbA_{1c} value of 7.5% was associated with a heightened risk of adverse events (Figure 4.8). These results reinforce the finding of increased mortality (HR 1.22, 95% CI 1.01–1.46), noticed in the intensive treatment arm (target HbA_{1c} <6.0% vs.7.0–7.9%) of the ACCORD trial.

HR for all-cause mortality in people given insulin-based regimens (2834 deaths) versus those given combination oral agents (2035) was 1.49 (95% CI 1.39–1.59). Whether this further heightened risk of death relates to the intensification of glucose control with insulin therapy remains unclear and needs further investigation.

In contrast, researchers from the ADVANCE and the VADT studies failed to show any increase in mortality in the intensively treated patients. These trials also failed to demonstrate that achievement of

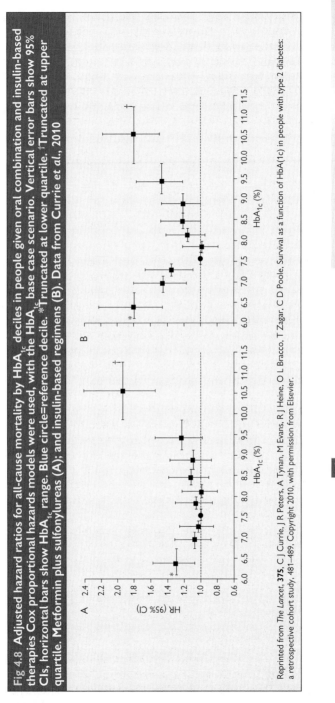

Fig 4.8 Adjusted hazard ratios for all-cause mortality by HbA$_{1c}$ deciles in people given oral combination and insulin-based therapies Cox proportional hazards models were used, with the HbA$_{1c}$ base case scenario. Vertical error bars show 95% CIs, horizontal bars show HbA$_{1c}$ range. Blue circle=reference decile. *Truncated at lower quartile. †Truncated at upper quartile. Metformin plus sulfonylureas (A); and insulin-based regimens (B). Data from Currie et al., 2010

Reprinted from *The Lancet*, **375**, C J Currie, J R Peters, A Tynan, M Evans, R J Heine, O L Bracco, T Zagar, C D Poole, Survival as a function of HbA(1c) in people with type 2 diabetes: a retrospective cohort study, 481–489, Copyright 2010, with permission from Elsevier.

good glycaemic control was associated with reduction of cardiovascular risk. The VADT researchers (2009) suggest that intensive blood glucose control early on (closer to a person's diagnosis of diabetes) may be more helpful in preventing cardiovascular problems than intensifying control later. NICE recognizes this and indicates a target HbA$_{1c}$ of 6.5% in the initial years after diagnosis of diabetes (first two treatment steps) and a target of less than 7.5% thereafter.

4.7.3 Combination of OHA and insulin therapy

All OADs require significant circulating insulin to be effective and their actions progressively reduce with declining beta-cell function as the disease progress. On the other hand, insulin therapy alone often results in increasing insulin resistance due to weight gain, resulting in need for larger doses of insulin. Combinations of insulin with OHAs therefore may result in improved efficacy but with potentially less weight gain. Indeed, in UKPDS, combination therapy of insulin and either metformin or sulfonylurea improved glycaemic control over insulin treatment alone (Wright et al., 2002). One meta-analysis reports better HbA$_{1c}$ and fasting glucose profile with combination therapy of insulin and sulfonylurea (Johnson et al., 1996). Analysis by Yki-Jarvinen (2001) reports modest but better glycaemic control, reduced insulin doses and weight gain with combination therapy of insulin and metformin.

4.7.4 Regimes of insulin in type 2 diabetes

There are very few randomized trials to enable decisions regarding choice of appropriate insulin regimens in diabetes. Therefore, many insulin treatment regimens have been tried but the most common regimes used are often in combination with OADs, especially metformin:

- Once-daily intermediate-acting (such as isophane insulin) or basal insulin (such as insulin glargine) regime in combination with an OHA (most commonly metformin). The insulin is most frequently injected at night, with the intention of reducing increased overnight hepatic glucose production
- Twice-daily intermediate-acting (e.g. isophane insulin) or once or twice daily insulin analogues (e.g. insulin detemir or insulin glargine)
- Twice-a-day pre-mixed human insulins or insulin analogues of variable proportion (most commonly 30% short-acting and 70% intermediate-acting)
- The basal-bolus regime of multiple injections of prandial rapid acting insulin analogues or short-acting soluble insulin with once-daily injection of intermediate or long-acting human insulin or insulin analogues
- The insulin regime should be tailored to the patient's individual circumstances.

For patients with type 2 diabetes, once-per-day basal insulin often gives adequate glycaemic control, and insulin glargine and detemir have equal efficacy for glycaemic control but reduced risk of overnight hypogly-caemia compared to isophane insulin (NPH) (Yki-Järvinen *et al.*, 2000; Rosenstock *et al.*, 2001; Horvath *et al.*, 2007). When patients have post-prandial hyperglycaemic peaks, an addition of short/rapid-acting insulin or changing to pre-mixed twice-a-day insulin regime may be beneficial.

4.7.4.1 Prandial or basal insulin first?
Traditionally, basal insulin has been the most commonly commenced first insulin in patients with type 2 diabetes. However, Monnier *et al.* (2007) demonstrated a 3-step decline in glucose homeostasis. First, patients exhibit a loss of post-prandial glycaemic control, which is followed by a decline in control of pre-breakfast and post-breakfast periods, culminating with sustained nocturnal hyperglycaemia, which results in fasting hyperglycaemia. Even at overall HbA_{1c} <7.3%, post-prandial glucose excursions can contribute to fluctuating levels of glycaemia (Monnier *et al.*, 2003). These findings suggest that earlier initiation of prandial insulin, prior to basal insulin, may be the appro-priate insulin to initiate, and followed by the addition of basal insulin.

4.7.4.2 Which insulin regime?
Two studies looked at insulin initiation strategies for type 2 patients on oral therapy, i.e. the AT.LANTUS study (Davies M *et al.*, 2005) with insulin glargine, and the 4-T study with insulin detemir (Levemir®) (2009).

The Treating To Target in Type 2 Diabetes study (4-T) study compared three different insulin strategies (biphasic insulin aspart twice daily, prandial insulin aspart three times daily, or basal insulin detemir once daily) in 708 patients with type 2 diabetes who were suboptimally controlled with metformin and a sulfonylurea. At the end of 3 years, there was no difference in the median HbA_{1c} in the 3 groups (7.1%, 6.8% and 6.9% respectively); however, a higher % of patients in the basal and prandial groups achieve HbA_{1c} less than 6.5 when compared to the biphasic group (42%, 45% and 31.9% respec-tively). Rates of hypoglycaemia were lowest in the basal group (1.7). The prandial group had the highest rates of hypoglycaemia (5.7) along with highest increase in mean weight (3.6kg for basal, 5.7kg for premixed insulin and 6.4kg for the prandial insulin) (Figure 4.9).

The results of the 4-T support the initial addition of basal insulin to oral therapy, with subsequent intensification to a basal-prandial regimen, consistent with consensus recommendations.

Although the 4 T study showed that basal or prandial insulin regi-mens provided better glycaemic control when added to oral therapy vs. adding to a biphasic (aspart-based) regimen, total insulin dose was high-est in the basal group (88 U), prandial insulin use was higher in the basal group (51 vs 28 U in the biphasic group) and most patients eventually received more complex insulin regimens irrespective of initial therapy.

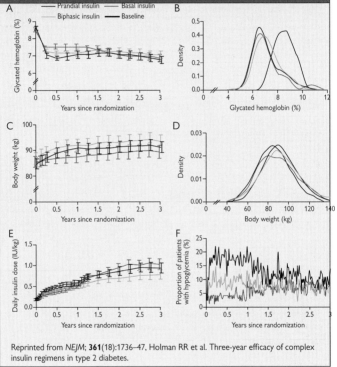

Fig 4.9 Primary and secondary outcomes at 3 Years. Panel A shows median levels of glycated hemoglobin in the three study groups, with a kernel-density plot of the distribution of values for patients in each group at 3 years, as compared with the distribution of values for all patients at baseline, shown in Panel B. Panel C shows mean body weight, with a kernel-density plot of the distribution of values for patients in each group at 3 years, as compared with the distribution of values for all patients at baseline, shown in Panel D. Panel E shows median insulin doses. Panel F shows the proportions of patients in the three study groups reporting grade 2 or grade 3 hypoglycemic events over time. The I bars indicate 95% confidence intervals.

Reprinted from *NEJM*; **361**(18):1736–47, Holman RR et al. Three-year efficacy of complex insulin regimens in type 2 diabetes.

AT.LANTUS (Davies M et al., 2008) shows that initiation of once-daily insulin glargine with OADs results in significant reduction of HbA$_{1c}$ with a low risk of hypoglycaemia. The greater reduction in HbA$_{1c}$ was seen in patients randomized to the patient-driven algorithm on 1 or >1 OAD.

It has so far not been proven that long-acting insulin analogues (LAIAs) have an advantage over conventional human insulin in the treatment of patients with type 2 diabetes. In a meta-analysis by

Fig 4.10 (a) Differences (with 95% CI) between long-acting analogues and NPH insulin in the effects on HbA$_{1c}$ at endpoint. (b) Differences (with 95% CI) between long-acting analogues and NPH insulin in the incidence of any, severe, symptomatic, and nocturnal hypoglycaemia. Data from Monami et al., 2008

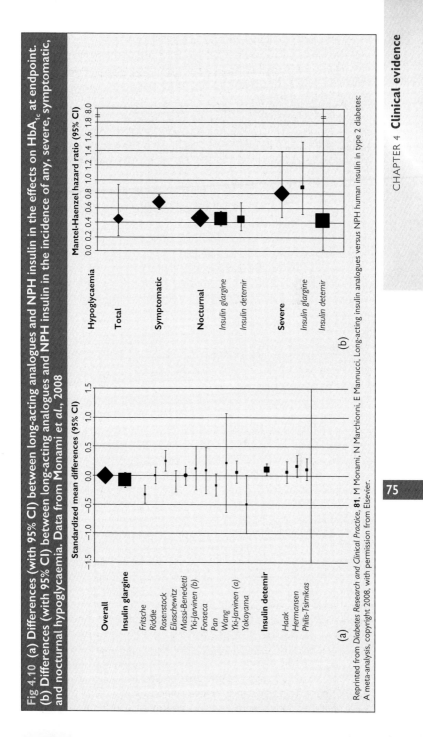

Reprinted from Diabetes Research and Clinical Practice, **81**, M Monami, N Marchionni, E Mannucci, Long-acting insulin analogues versus NPH human insulin in type 2 diabetes: A meta-analysis, copyright 2008, with permission from Elsevier.

Monami *et al.* (2008) comparing long acting insulin analogues versus NPH human insulin in type 2 diabetes, the use of the former does not seem to provide better glycaemic control in comparison with NPH insulin, but it reduces the risk of nocturnal and symptomatic hypoglycaemia (Figure 4.10a,b). This analysis also concludes that insulin detemir but not glargine could be associated with a smaller weight gain than NPH insulin. NICE still recommends beginning with human NPH insulin as the first step in insulin initiation.

4.7.4.3 Side effects

Weight gain and hypoglycaemia are among the well-known side effects of insulin therapy. In the UKPDS, obese patients treated with insulin gained 4 kg of weight during 6 years (compared to 1 kg and 6 kg weight gain with metformin and sulfonylurea, respectively). However, the majority of weight gain with insulin therapy is attributed to cor-rection of glycosuria (Nikkilä *et al.*, 1999), whilst basal metabolic rate and energy intake remain unchanged. Generally, improved glycaemic control is related to more frequent hypoglycaemia but combination therapy of insulin and metformin is associated with relatively less hypoglycaemia (Yki-Jarvinen *et al.*, 1999).

4.8 Diabetes treatments: cancer risk and prognosis

There is increasing evidence from epidemiological studies that supports an association between the incidence and prognosis of certain types of cancers and diabetes. Though a number of possible mechanisms have been described (hyperglycemia, hyperinsulinaemia, and inflammation), it is now believed that there is no causal relationship and the association is due to common predisposing risk factors (*viz.* obesity, smoking and alcohol consumption) that they share. Recently, some of the diabetes treatments have come under intense scrutiny for their potential to influ-ence the incidence of cancer or affect cancer prognosis.

In spite of the introduction of newer anti-diabetes agents, met-formin remains the first-line therapeutic agent for the treatment of type 2 diabetes. In several observational studies (comparing other glucose lowering therapies) treatment with metformin has been associated with a reduced risk of cancer (Monami *et al.*, 2009; Currie *et al.*, 2009) or cancer mortality (Landman *et al.*, 2010). These results have to be cautiously interpreted as metformin is used early in the treatment of diabetes and patients with advanced age, kidney and liver disease would not have been prescribed metformin.

Another recent observational study demonstrated that metformin treatment was associated with a better response in patients with early stage breast cancer receiving neoadjuvant therapy (Cazzaniga *et al.*, 2009). A clinical trial is ongoing to further evaluate the potential effect of metformin on breast cancer prognosis (as measured by Ki67 index).

Similar findings of higher cancer risk have been reported from observational studies among patients with type 2 diabetes treated with sulfonylureas. However, due to the low incidence of cancer in these studies further associations with specific cancer sites was not possible and it was difficult to determine whether the findings reflected excess cancer among users of sulfonylureas. There have been no reports of meglitinides or incretin-based therapies on human cancer incidence.

Whilst thiazolidinediones have recently been surrounded by controversy over their cardiovascular safety, in vitro studies with PPARγ agonists attribute several anti cancer properties like inhibition of cell growth, differentiation and ability to induce apoptosis. These findings are contradicted, however, by the findings of increased tumorigenesis in rodent studies and the possibility of increased risk of bladder cancer in human studies. There is currently no robust human data available on cancer risk associated with thiazolidinediones.

Recent epidemiological studies have examined the possible association between the use of insulin glargine and increased risk of cancer. The findings from these studies have been widely debated. Caveats to the interpretation of these results lies in the fact that insulin glargine is the most frequently prescribed insulin in England, and it is more commonly prescribed in patients with longer duration of type 2 diabetes and in people with other co-morbidities, in whom other comparator medications cannot be prescribed.

The plausible mechanisms postulated for insulin induced carcinogenesis include a direct action of the analogue insulins or their active metabolites. Insulin glargine has been shown to have a much higher affinity for the IGF-1 receptor, and a higher mitogenic potency, than human insulin or other analogues (Kurtzhals, 2000; Liefvendahl, 2008; Shukla, 2009). It has been demonstrated that knockdown of IGF-1 receptors abolished the proliferation of malignant cell lines induced by insulin glargine. Indirect mechanisms involve interactions of various signaling molecules (e.g. glucagon, adiponectin, or IGFBPs) whose levels or activity are influenced by administration of insulin.

Four retrospective observational studies published in 2009 (Hemkens et al., Jonasson et al., Colhoun et al. and Currie et al.) have suggested the possibility of an association between use of insulin glargine and cancer. However the German study by Hemkens et al. (2009) which initially reported a higher incidence of cancer with the use of human insulins has been criticized for methodological aberrations: patients treated with insulin glargine were considered to have greater frailty and co-morbidities (including cancer) and may have had lower insulin doses and higher glucose levels deliberately. Also, patients with both type 1 and type 2 diabetes were included and therefore will have had treatment with insulin combinations other than insulin glargine. The Swedish study by Jonasson reports greater risk for breast cancer in a sub-population using insulin glargine only vs. non-insulin glargine users, but the risk disappears when insulin glargine is used in combination with other insulins. Notably, the study does not indicate greater cancer risk with increasing insulin glargine dose.

At the same time, the results of the longest randomized trial comparing human insulin NPH and glargine in type 2 diabetes was published, reporting no difference in cancer risk (Rosenstock et al., 2009).

In a recent case-control study of type 2 diabetic patients, during a median follow-up of 76 months, 112 cases of incident cancer were compared to 370 matched controls. A significantly higher mean daily dose of insulin glargine was observed in cases than in controls (0.24 [0.10; 0.39] vs. 0.16 [0.12; 0.24] IU/day*kg, $p=0.036$). The incidence of cancer was associated with a dose of insulin glargine ˇ 0.3 IU/kg/day even after adjusting for Charlson co-morbidity score, other types of insulin administration, and metformin exposure (OR 5.43, 95% CI [2.18; 13.53]; $p<0.001$). This study by Mannucci et al. (2010) highlights the possibility of association between occurrence of cancer and higher doses of insulin glargine but the >0.3 IU/kg/day was an entirely arbitrary cut off figure open to significant criticism.

Epidemiological studies cannot provide definite conclusions about the association of insulin and cancer. To comprehensively evaluate and solve the current controversies further investigations will be needed. The International Study of Insulin and Cancer (ISICA) is one such study that aims mainly to assess the association of breast cancer with the use of individual insulins such as the analogues (glargine, lispro, and aspart) and human insulin formulations (isophane and regular human insulin), compared with non-insulin use in patients with diabetes. This is a case-control study currently underway across UK, France and Canada, the results of which are expected in mid-2012.

4.9 **Conclusions**

Whilst established and newer agents appear to increase the armamentarium of the clinician involved in care for the patients with type 2 diabetes, the ultimate therapy remains elusive. Such a therapy would be a once-daily oral or injectable preparation, with long-term glycaemic efficacy, which therefore reduces the otherwise inexorable decline of beta-cell function and, most important, is safe. Indeed we remain unsure of the timing and methodology of insulin therapy. An additional benefit would be a reduction of cardiovascular risk, which to date has not been demonstrated conclusively for any therapy for type 2 diabetes. The incretin-based treatments hold promise in offering a viable alternative to the existing choices but are yet to demonstrate their cardiovascular and overall safety in long term trials. The current evidence suggests potential carcinogenic effects of analogue insulins and warrant further studies.

References

Brown JB, Conner C, Nichols GA (2010) Secondary failure rate of metformin monotherapy in clinical practice. *Diabet Care* **33**: 501–506.

Cazzaniga M, Bonanni B, Guerrieri-Gonzaga A, Decensi A (2009) Is it time to test metformin in breast cancer clinical trials? *Cancer Epidemiol Biomarkers Prev* **18**: 701–5.

Colhoun HM; SDRN Epidemiology Group (2009) Use of insulin glargine and cancer incidence in Scotland: a study from the Scottish Diabetes Research Network Epidemiology Group. *Diabetologia* **52**: 1755–65.

Currie CJ, Peters JR, Tynan A, *et al.* (2010) Survival as a function of HbA(1c) in people with type 2 diabetes: a retrospective cohort study. *Lancet* **375**: 481–9.

Currie CJ, Poole CD, Gale EA (2009) The influence of glucose-lowering therapies on cancer risk in type 2 diabetes. *Diabetologia* **52**: 1766–77.

Davies M, Lavalle-González F, Storms F, Gomis R; AT.LANTUS Study Group (2008) Initiation of insulin glargine therapy in type 2 diabetes subjects sub optimally controlled on oral antidiabetic agents: results from the AT.LANTUS trial. *Diabetes Obes Metab* **10**: 387–99.

Diabetes Control and Complications Trial Research Group (1993) The effect of intensive treatment of diabetes on the development and progression of long-term complications in insulin-dependent diabetes mellitus. *N Engl J Med* **329**: 977.

Duckkworth W, Abraira C, Moritz T, *et al.*, on behalf of the VADT Investigators (2009) Glucose control and vascular complications in Veterans with type 2 diabetes. *N Engl J Med* **360**: 129–39.

Hemkens LG, Grouven U, Bender R (2009) Risk of malignancies in patients with diabetes treated with human insulin or insulin analogues: a cohort study. *Diabetologia* **52**: 1732–44.

Holman RR, Farmer AJ, Davies MJ, Levy JC, Darbyshire JL, Keenan JF, Paul SK; 4-T Study Group. (2010) Three-year efficacy of complex insulin regimens in type 2 diabetes. *N Engl J Med* **361**: 1736–47.

Horvath K, Jeitler K, Berghold A, *et al.* (2007) Long-acting insulin analogues versus NPH insulin (human isophane insulin) for type 2 diabetes mellitus. *Cochrane Database Syst Rev*: CD005613.

Hu FB, Stampfer MJ, Solomon CG, *et al.* (2001) The impact of diabetes mellitus on mortality from all causes and coronary heart disease in women: 20 years of follow-up. *Arch Intern Med* **161**: 1717–1723.

Inzucchi SE, Bergenstal RM, Buse JB *et al.* (2012) Management of hyperglycaemia in type 2 diabetes: a patient-centered approach. Position statement of the American Diabetes Association (ADA) and the European Association for the Study of Diabetes (EASD). *Diabetologia* **55**: 1577–1596.

Jonasson JM, Ljung R, Talback M (2009) Insulin glargine use and short-term incidence of malignancies-a population-based follow-up study in Sweden. *Diabetologia* **52**: 1745–54.

Kahn SE, Haffner SM, Heise MA, *et al.* (2007) Glycemic durability of rosiglitazone, metformin, or glyburide monotherapy. *N Engl J Med* **355**: 2427–43.

Kurtzhals P, Schaffer L, Sørensen A, Kristensen C, Jonassen I, Schmid C, Trub T (2000) Correlations of receptor binding and metabolic and mitogenic potencies of insulin analogs designed for clinical use. *Diabetes* **49**: 999–1005.

Landman GW, Kleefstra N, van Hateren KJ, Groenier KH, Gans RO, Bilo HJ (2010) Metformin associated with lower cancer mortality in type 2 diabetes: ZODIAC- 16. *Diabet Care* **33**: 322–326.

Mannucci E, Monami M, Balzi D, *et al.* (2010) Doses of insulin and its analogues and cancer occurrence in insulin-treated type 2 diabetic patients. *Diabet Care* **33**: 1997–2003.

Monami M, Lamanna C, Balzi D, Marchionni N, Mannucci E (2009) Sulphonylureas and cancer: a case-control study. *Acta Diabetol*; **46**: 279–284.

Monami M, Marchionni N, Mannucci E (2008) Long-acting insulin analogues versus NPH human insulin in type 2 diabetes: a meta-analysis. *Diabetes Reserach and Clinical Practice* **81**: 184–189.

Monnier L, Colette C, Dunseath GJ, *et al.* (2007) The loss of postprandial glycemic control precedes stepwise deterioration of fasting with worsening diabetes. *Diabet Care* **30**: 263–9.

Nathan DM (2002) Clinical practice. Initial management of glycemia in type 2 diabetes mellitus. *N Engl J Med* **347**: 1342–9.

Nathan DM, Buse JB, Davidson MB, *et al.* (2009) Consensus statement update; Medical Management of Hyperglycaemia in Type 2 diabetes: a consensus algorithm for the initiation and adjustment of therapy. *Diabetologia* **52**: 17–30.

Nissen SE, Wolski K. (2007) Effect of rosiglitazone on the risk of myocardial infarction and death from cardiovascular causes. *N Engl J Med* **356**: 2457–2471.

Nissen SE, Wolski K (2010) Rosiglitazone revisited: an updated meta-analysis of risk for myocardial infarction and cardiovascular mortality. *Arch Intern Med* **170**: 1191–1201.

Pantalone KM, Kattan MW, Yu C, *et al.* (2010) The risk of overall mortality in patients with type 2 diabetes receiving glipizide, glyburide, or glimepiride monotherapy: a retrospective analysis. *Diabet Care* **33**: 1224–9.

Pocock SJ, Smeeth L (2009) Insulin glargine and malignancy: an unwarranted alarm. *Lancet* **374**: 511–13.

Ray KK, Seshasai SR, Wijesuriya S, *et al.* (2009) Effect of intensive control of glucose on cardiovascular outcomes and death in patients with diabetes mellitus: a meta-analysis of randomised controlled trials. *Lancet* **373**: 1765–72.

Rosenstock J, Schwartz SL, Clark CM Jr, *et al.* (2001) Basal insulin therapy in type 2 diabetes: 28-week comparison of insulin glargine (HOE 901) and NPH insulin. *Diabet Care* **24**: 631.

Saenz A, Fernandez-Esteban I, Mataix A *et al.* (2005) Metformin monotherapy for type 2 diabetes mellitus, : *Cochrane Database Syst Rev* **4**: Issue 3. Art. No.: CD002966. DOI: 10.1002/146S1858.CD002966.pub3.

Stratton IM, Adler AI, Neil HA, *et al.* (2000) Association of glycaemia with macrovascular and microvascular complications of type 2 diabetes (UKPDS 35): prospective observational study. *BMJ* **321**: 405–12.

The Action to Control Cardiovascular Risk in Diabetes Study Group (2008) Effects of intensive glucose-lowering in type 2 diabetes. *New Engl J Med* **358**: 2545–59.

The ADVANCE Collaborative Group (2008) Intensive blood glucose control and vascular outcomes in patients with type 2 diabetes. *N Engl J Med* **358**: 2560–72.

UKPDS (UK Prospective Diabetes Study Group) (1998) Effect of intensive blood-glucose control with metformin on complications in overweight patients with type 2 diabetes (UKPDS 34). *Lancet* **352**: 854.

UKPDS (1998) UKPDS 24: A 6 year, randomized, controlled trial comparing sulphonylurea, insulin and metformin therapy in patients with newly diagnosed type 2 diabetes that could not be controlled with diet therapy. *Ann Intern Med* **128**: 165–75.

Suggested reading

Davies M, Lavalle-González F, Storms F, Gomis R; AT.LANTUS Study Group (2008) Initiation of insulin glargine therapy in type 2 diabetes subjects suboptimally controlled on oral antidiabetic agents: results from the AT.LANTUS trial. *Diabetes Obes Metab* May; **10**: 387–99.

Giovannucci E, Harlan DM, Archer MC, *et al.* (2010) Diabetes and cancer: a consensus report. *Diabetes Care* **33**: 1674–85.

Holman RR, Farmer AJ, Davies MJ, Levy JC, Darbyshire JL, Keenan JF, Paul SK; 4-T Study Group (2010) Three-year efficacy of complex insulin regimens in type 2 diabetes. *N Engl J Med* **361**: 1736–47.

Nathan DM, Buse JB, Davidson MB, *et al.* (2009) Consensus statement update; medical management of hyperglycaemia in Type 2 diabetes: a consensus algorithm for the initiation and adjustment of therapy. *Diabetologia* **52**: 17–30.

Chapter 5

Multiple cardiovascular risk intervention

Miles Fisher

Key points

- Cardiovascular disease is a common cause of morbidity and mortality in people with type 2 diabetes. Some guidelines define diabetes as a coronary heart disease equivalent, requiring multiple cardiovascular risk factor reduction
- The treatment of hyperglycaemia in type 2 diabetes reduces cardiovascular events, and on long-term follow up reduces cardiovascular and total mortality. Metformin and pioglitazone have advantages in subgroups of patients
- There is a large evidence base for the treatment of hypertension in people with type 2 diabetes, using multiple antihypertensive drugs, and for the use of statins. The results of studies of other lipid-regulating drugs have been disappointing
- Benefits of other methods to reduce cardiovascular risk, such as antiplatelet drugs and antioxidants, have yet to be established in people with type 2 diabetes.

83

'Diabetes is a state of premature cardiovascular death which is associated with chronic hyperglycaemia and may also be associated with blindness and renal failure.'

Miles Fisher, British Diabetic Association meeting Dublin, 1996.

5.1 Introduction

5.1.1 Pathophysiology of heart disease in diabetes

Cardiovascular disease is a common cause of morbidity and mortality in people with diabetes. Coronary heart disease frequently presents

Table 5.1 Risk factors for coronary heart disease and myocardial infarction in the UKPDS (UKPDS 23)

Coronary artery disease	Fatal or non-fatal myocardial infarction	Fatal myocardial infarction
Raised LDL cholesterol	Raised LDL cholesterol	Diastolic blood pressure
Low HDL cholesterol	Diastolic blood pressure	Raised LDL cholesterol
HbA$_{1c}$	Smoking	HbA$_{1c}$
Systolic blood pressure	Low HDL cholesterol	
Smoking	HbA$_{1c}$	

Reproduced from *British Medical Journal*, Turner, R.C., Millns, H., Neil, H.A.W. *et al*, **316**, 823–8, 1998 with permission from BMJ Publishing Group Ltd.

as an acute coronary syndrome, and diabetic patients have more silent myocardial ischaemia, which may be related to diabetic cardiovascular autonomic neuropathy. Severe autonomic neuropathy also causes a reduced exercise capacity, resting tachycardia, and postural hypotension, but is fortunately rare. There is a 'diabetic cardiomyopathy' that can impair systolic emptying or diastolic filling of the left ventricle, and along with coronary heart disease may contribute to the high prevalence of chronic heart failure in people with diabetes.

5.1.2 Risk factors for coronary heart disease in diabetes

In the United Kingdom Prospective Diabetes Study (UKPDS) hypertension, dyslipidaemia, hyperglycaemia and smoking were independent risk factors for coronary events, indicating the potential for risk factor intervention in people with type 2 diabetes (Table 5.1).

There are now multiple therapies that can be used to reduce cardiovascular risk in people with diabetes (Box 5.1). However, if we are going to obtain the greatest benefit and wish to reduce polypharmacy we should concentrate on the use of strategies that have a proven evidence base.

5.2 Management of hyperglycaemia to reduce cardiovascular risk

5.2.1 UKPDS and metformin

The UKPDS tested the hypothesis that tight glycaemia control in type 2 diabetes would reduce microvascular and macrovascular complications. The principal comparisons were between patients that received conventional treatment and patients that received intensive

> **Box 5.1 Interventions to reduce cardiovascular risk in people with type 2 diabetes**
>
> Treatment of hyperglycaemia
> - Intensive blood glucose control
> - Additional benefits of metformin, pioglitazone
>
> Treatment of dyslipidaemia
> - Statins
> - Additional benefits of high-dose atorvastatin
>
> Treatment of hypertension
> - Multiple antihypertensive drugs
> - Additional benefits of ACE inhibitors, angiotensin II receptor antagonists
>
> Antiplatelet drugs
> - Aspirin and/or clopidogrel for established cardiovascular disease

treatment based on therapy with a sulfonylurea or insulin. A small subgroup of overweight patients was also randomized to metformin.

Tight control reduced microvascular endpoints, in particular the need for photocoagulation for diabetic retinopathy. There was a statistically insignificant reduction in myocardial infarctions. The main side effects of sulfonylureas were weight gain and hypoglycaemia, and there was no evidence of adverse cardiovascular effects.

Metformin significantly reduced myocardial infarctions and all-cause mortality in the overweight patients, which could not be explained by any differences in HbA_{1c}, suggesting that benefits were due to some other effect of metformin.

Most of the patients in UKPDS were followed in post-trial monitoring for a further 10 years. No attempt was made to maintain previously assigned therapies and glycaemic control in the groups rapidly converged, so that between-group differences in HbA_{1c} were lost after the first year. In the group who had received metformin as initial therapy, significant reductions in myocardial infarction and all-cause mortality persisted. In the group who had received sulfonylureas or insulin as initial intensive therapy, significant reductions in myocardial infarctions and all-cause mortality emerged—a so-called 'legacy' effect.

5.2.2 **Pioglitazone and the PROactive study**

The thiazolidinediones rosiglitazone and pioglitazone have potentially beneficial effects on several cardiovascular risk factors (Box 5.2). Glitazones cause weight gain, and the effects on lipids are significantly different; pioglitazone reduces triglycerides and increases

Box 5.2 Effects of glitazones on cardiovascular risk factors

Potentially beneficial:

• improved glycaemic control
• reduced blood pressure
• reduced microalbuminuria
• reduced C-reactive protein
• reduced small dense LDL (especially pioglitazone)
• increased HDL cholesterol (especially pioglitazone)
• reduced triglycerides (pioglitazone).

Potentially adverse:

• weight gain
• increased total and LDL cholesterol (rosiglitazone).

high density lipoprotein (HDL) cholesterol whereas rosiglitazone increases total and low density lipoprotein (LDL) cholesterol.

Glitazones cause fluid retention via renal mechanisms. In a patient with early left ventricular systolic dysfunction, or diastolic dysfunction, this fluid retention can unmask heart failure. Glitazones are contra-indicated in patients with chronic heart failure.

The PROactive study (PROspective pioglitAzone Clinical Trial In macroVascular Events) examined the effects of pioglitazone on cardiovascular events in patients with type 2 diabetes and existing cardiovascular disease. There was a statistically insignificant reduction of 10% in the primary endpoint, which comprised disease endpoints and procedural endpoints. A main secondary endpoint of cardiovascular death, myocardial infarction or stroke, was significantly reduced by 16%. Subgroup analysis of patients who had a previous myocardial infarction or strokes showed further reductions in myocardial infarctions and strokes, respectively.

Meta-analysis of cardiovascular events in patients treated with pioglitazone has demonstrated significant reductions in cardiovascular events.

5.2.3 Rosiglitazone meta-analysis and the RECORD study

The effects of rosiglitazone on cardiovascular outcomes remain controversial. A meta-analysis was performed of trials where rosiglitazone was given for at least 24 weeks, with a comparable group not receiving rosiglitazone, and the outcome data collected for myocardial infarction and death from cardiovascular causes. In the rosiglitazone group there were 86 myocardial infarctions in 15,560 subjects, and in the comparator group there were 72 myocardial infarctions in 12,283 subjects, giving an odds ratio of 1.43 for myocardial infarction (95%

confidence interval 1.03–1.99; $p = 0.03$) with an insignificant increase in cardiovascular deaths. Similar results have been found in an updated meta-analysis from the same authors, and in meta-analyses performed by the Federal Drug Administration (FDA).

The Rosiglitazone Evaluated for Cardiac Outcomes and Regulation of glycaemia in Diabetes (RECORD) study was prospectively established to examine the cardiovascular effects of rosiglitazone. An interim analysis was published following the Nissen meta-analysis, which highlighted major deficiencies in study design. The study was open label and not double blind, and was a 'non-inferiority' study. The primary event rate was much lower than predicted. When RECORD was completed there were no significant differences between the rosiglitazone group and the control group regarding myocardial infarction and death from cardiovascular causes, but an increase in these could not be excluded.

To try and definitively answer safety concerns about rosiglitazone a double-blind trial comparing rosiglitazone with pioglitazone in diabetic patients with vascular disease or high vascular risk was started. In late 2010 the European Medicines Agency recommended the suspension of marketing authorization for rosiglitazone across Europe and this has been withdrawn from clinical use.

5.2.4 **Other anti-diabetic drugs**

Meta-analysis of the effects of acarbose in patients with type 2 diabetes has given conflicting results. One meta-analysis suggested a reduction in cardiovascular events, whereas a Cochrane review suggested no evidence of any benefit for mortality and morbidity.

Of the newer antidiabetic drugs DPP-4 inhibitors reduce HbA_{1c}, are weight neutral, but have little discernable effect on cardiovascular risk markers. Glucagon-like peptide-1 (GLP-1) receptor agonists reduce HbA_{1c} and weight, with slight but significant reductions in blood pressure, and some improvement in the lipid profile associated with weight loss. Sodium glucose co-transporter 2 inhibitors (SGLT2 inhibitors) also reduce HbA_{1c}, weight, and blood pressure, which may be related to renal sodium loss. Cardiovascular safety and/or end-point trials are currently in progress with several DPP-4 inhibitors, GLP-1 receptor agonists, and SGLT2 inhibitors.

5.2.5 **Glycaemic targets**

In the UKPDS the mean HbA_{1c} concentration in the intensive treatment group was 7.0%. Two important large multi-centre studies were set up to examine if a lower target HbA_{1c} would reduce cardiovascular events.

• The Action in Diabetes and Vascular disease: preterAx and diamicroN-MR Controlled Evaluation (ADVANCE) study aimed to obtain a target HbA_{1c} of 6.5% in the intensive group, and this was achieved three years into the study. There was a significant reduction in microvascular events with more intensive therapy in ADVANCE, but no significant effect, either beneficial or harmful, on macrovascular events or mortality. Weight gain and hypoglycaemia were not common in ADVANCE.

• The Action to Control Cardiovascular Risk in Diabetes (ACCORD) study aimed to reduce HbA_{1c} rapidly to non-diabetic levels. The target HbA_{1c} of less than 6.0% was not reached because of severe hypoglycaemia and marked weight gain, and a level of 6.5% was obtained by 6 months. The study was stopped early because of an increase in total mortality in the intensive treatment group. To date the investigators have failed to satisfactorily explain the increased mortality. As several of the deaths were sudden or unexpected, undetected hypoglycaemia provoking arrhythmias is a possible explanation.

Several meta-analyses have been performed which have included data from UKPDS, ADVANCE and ACCORD. Significant reductions in myocardial infarctions and coronary events have been observed, with no significant effect on strokes or cardiovascular mortality (Figure 5.1). The target HbA_{1c} for the prevention of cardiovascular disease in diabetes should be less than 7.0% and not lower than 6.5%.

Fig 5.1 Probablity of events of non-fatal myocardial infarction with intensive glucose-lowering versus standard treatment (Ray et al., 2009)

	Intensive treatment/ standard treatment		Weight of study size	Odds ratio (95% CI)	Odds ratio (95% CI)
	Participants	Events			
UKPDS	3071/1549	221/141	21.8%		0.78 (0.62–0.98)
PROactive	2605/2633	119/144	18.0%		0.83 (0.64–1.06)
ADVANCE	5571/5569	153/156	21.9%		0.98 (0.78–1.23)
VADT	892/899	64/78	9.4%		0.81 (0.58–1.15)
ACCORD	5128/5123	186/235	28.9%		0.78 (0.64–0.95)
Overall	17267/15773	743/754	100%		0.83 (0.75–0.93)

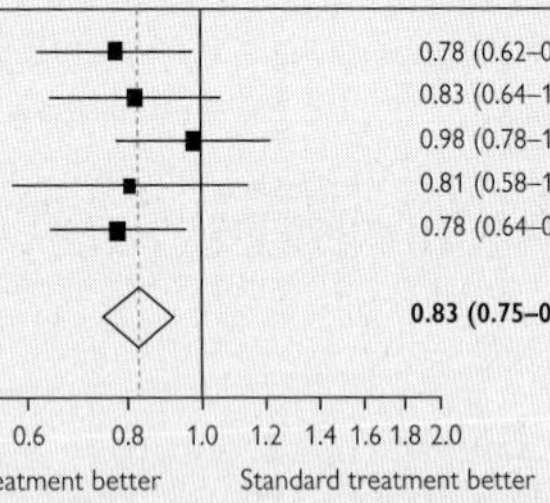

0.4   0.6   0.8   1.0   1.2 1.4 1.6 1.8 2.0
Intensive treatment better   Standard treatment better

Reprinted from *The Lancet*, **373**, Kausik K Ray, Sreenivasa Rao Kondapally Seshasai, Shanelle Wijesuriya, Rupa Sivakumaran, Sarah Nethercott, David Preiss, Sebhat Erqou, Naveed Sattar, Effect of intensive control of glucose on cardiovascular outcomes and death in patients with diabetes mellitus: a meta-analysis of randomised controlled trials, 1765–1772, 2009, with permission from Elsevier.

5.3 Management of dyslipidaemia to reduce cardiovascular risk

5.3.1 The dyslipidaemia of diabetes

Dyslipidaemia of type 2 diabetes and the metabolic syndrome consist of raised triglycerides and low HDL cholesterol. Total and LDL cholesterol concentrations tend not to be affected, although more of the LDL cholesterol is atherogenic small dense LDL cholesterol, and there are changes to some of the other lipid subfractions (Box 5.3). Of the available lipid-regulating drugs fibrates improve the lipid profile, reducing triglycerides and increasing HDL cholesterol, but there is conflicting evidence from clinical trials that this reduces cardiovascular events, and most of the evidence is for statins.

5.3.2 Statins

Initial statin trials were in patients with coronary heart disease and raised total cholesterol, using simvastatin and pravastatin. Subgroup analysis of diabetic subgroups demonstrated similar relative risk reductions for total mortality, cardiovascular mortality and major coronary events, and as the event rate was higher in people with diabetes the absolute risk reduction was greater.

Further statin trails were performed in subjects with 'normal' cholesterol concentrations, patients with other forms of vascular disease, and diabetic patients without known vascular disease, as well as studying other statins including atorvastatin. Several populations of diabetic patients have shown reductions in vascular events with statins compared to placebo (Box 5.4), but studies on patients with chronic renal failure, haemodialysis patients and patients with chronic heart failure have been negative.

5.3.3 Higher doses of statins

Epidemiological observations suggest that lower total or LDL cholesterol concentrations are associated with lower vascular events

---

Box 5.3 Diabetic dyslipidaemia

Increased
- triglycerides
- apolipoprotein B
- VLDL, especially VLDL1
- triglyceride-rich remnants
- small dense LDL
- postprandial lipaemia

Decreased
- HDL cholesterol, especially HDL2
- apolipoprotein A-1

Box 5.4 Statin use in diabetic subgroups

Statins of proven benefit

- Stable coronary disease with raised cholesterol
- Stable coronary disease with normal cholesterol
- Patients without known vascular disease ('primary prevention')
- Acute coronary syndromes
- Following coronary artery bypass surgery
- Following percutaneous coronary interventions
- Following stroke
- Early chronic kidney disease.

Statin studies negative

- Chronic renal failure
- Dialysis patients
- Chronic heart failure.

rates, leading to the hypothesis that higher doses of statins, leading to greater reductions in cholesterol, would lead to greater reductions in vascular events. Most of the comparisons have used high-dose atorvastatin, and further reductions in cardiovascular events have been demonstrated, including in diabetic subgroups (Figure 5.2). This has included in patients with acute coronary syndromes, objective

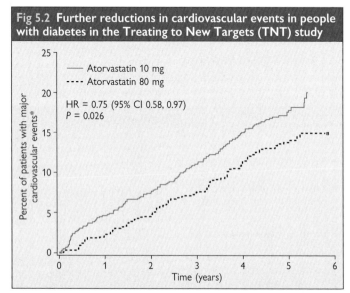

Fig 5.2 Further reductions in cardiovascular events in people with diabetes in the Treating to New Targets (TNT) study

Atorvastatin 10 mg
Atorvastatin 80 mg

HR = 0.75 (95% CI 0.58, 0.97)
P = 0.026

Percent of patients with major cardiovascular events*

Time (years)

evidence of coronary heart disease on angiography, and following coronary revascularization procedures.

Reductions have been in non-fatal events, so that there has not been any further reduction in total or cardiovascular mortality. The main side effects of the higher doses have been an increase in abnormalities of liver function tests.

5.3.4 Meta-analysis of cholesterol lowering

The Cholesterol Treatment Trialists' (CTT) Collaborators performed a meta-analysis of cholesterol-lowering therapy in 18 686 people with diabetes in 14 randomized trials of statins. There was a 9% reduction in all-cause mortality per mmol/L reduction in LDL cholesterol, with a 21% reduction in major vascular events per mmol/L reduction in LDL cholesterol. There was some limited direct evidence of benefit in 1,466 people with type 1 diabetes in the HPS (Figure 5.3).

5.3.5 Cholesterol targets in diabetes

Present audit targets for cholesterol include a total cholesterol of 5 mmol/l, and an LDL cholesterol of 3 mmol/l. Evidence supports the

Fig 5.3 Effects on major vascular events per mmol/L reduction in LDL cholesterol by baseline factors in the CTT Collaboration

Groups	Events (%) Treatment	Events (%) Control	RR (CI)	Test for heterogenity or trend
Type of diabetes:				
Type 1 diabetes	147 (20·5%)	196 (26·2%)	0·79 (0·62–1·01)	χ^2_1=0·0; p=1·0
Type 2 diabetes	1318 (15·2%)	1586 (18·5%)	0·79 (0·72–0·87)	
Sex:				
Men	1082 (17·2%)	1332 (21·4%)	0·78 (0·71–0·86)	χ^2_1=0·1; p=0·7
Women	383 (12·4%)	450 (14·6%)	0·81 (0·67–0·97)	
Age (years):				
≤65	701 (13·1%)	898 (17·1%)	0·77 (0·68–0·87)	χ^2_1=0·5; p=0·5
>65	764 (18·9%)	884 (21·8%)	0·81 (0·71–0·92)	
Currently treated hypertension:				
Yes	1030 (16·3%)	1196 (19·1%)	0·82 (0·74–0·91)	χ^2_1=2·7; p=0·1
No	435 (14·2%)	586 (19·3%)	0·73 (0·63–0·85)	
Body-mass index:				
<25·0	276 (15·7%)	362 (20·4%)	0·78 (0·64–0·95)	χ^2_1=0·5; p=0·5
≥25·0–<30·0	639 (15·9%)	774 (19·8%)	0·77 (0·68–0·88)	
≥30.0	532 (15·1%)	628 (17·6%)	0·82 (0·71–0·95)	
Systolic blood pressure (mm Hg):				
<160	993 (15·0%)	1276 (19·1%)	0·76 (0·69–0·85)	χ^2_1=1·3; p=0·3
≥160	472 (17·1%)	505 (19·2%)	0·83 (0·71–0·96)	
Diastolic blood pressure (mm Hg):				
≤90	1176 (16·5%)	1417 (19·8%)	0·81 (0·73–0·89)	χ^2_1=1·7; p=0·2
>90	288 (12·9%)	364 (17·1%)	0·73 (0·61–0·87)	
Smoking status:				
Current smokers	266 (17·5%)	347 (22·5%)	0·78 (0·64–0·96)	χ^2_1=0·0; p=0·9
Non-smokers	1199 (15·2%)	1435 (18·5%)	0·79 (0·71–0·87)	
Estimated GFR (mL/min/1·73m²):				
<60	415 (20·6%)	477 (24·0%)	0·83 (0·71–0·97)	χ^2_1=2·9; p=0·09
≥60–<90	816 (15·5%)	961 (18·4%)	0·81 (0·72–0·91)	
≥90	194 (12·5%)	286 (18·7%)	0·65 (0·50–0·84)	
Predicted risk of major vascular event (per year):				
<4·5%	474 (8·4%)	631 (11·2%)	0·74 (0·64–0·85)	χ^2_1=1·8; p=0·2
≥4·5–8·0%	472 (23·2%)	540 (27·3%)	0·80 (0·66–0·96)	
≥8.0%	519 (30·5%)	611 (35·8%)	0·82 (0·70–0·95)	
All diabetes	**1465 (15·6%)**	**1782 (19·2%)**	**0·79 (0·74–0·84)**	

Global test for heterogeneity within subtotals: χ^2_{13}=13·9; p=0·4

0·5   1·0   1·5
Treatment better   Control better

■─ RR (99%CI)
◇ RR (95%CI)

Reprinted from *The Lancet*, **371**, Cholesterol Treatment Trialists' (CTT) Collaborators, Efficacy of cholesterol-lowering therapy in 18,686 people with diabetes in 14 randomised trials of statins: a meta-analysis, 117–125, 2008, with permission from Elsevier.

use of higher-dose statins to lower targets of 4 mmol/l total choles-terol and 2 mmol/l LDL cholesterol. This approach may not be cost effective in diabetic patients without known cardiovascular disease, but is strongly recommended for patients with established cardio-vascular disease, especially following acute coronary syndromes.

5.3.6 Other lipid-regulating drugs

Rosuvastatin is a newer, more potent statin, which causes greater reductions in total and LDL cholesterol. There are no endpoint trials to support rosuvastatin use in people with diabetes, and it should be con-sidered where diabetic patients have failed to reach targets with one of the other statins. In the Justification for the Use of statins in Prevention: an Intervention Trial Evaluating Rosuvastatin (JUPITER) study rosuvasta-tin reduced cardiovascular events in subjects with low LDL cholesterol levels and high concentrations of CRP, but people with diabetes were excluded. Indeed, there was a slight but significant increase in the devel-opment of new diabetes in subjects given rosuvastatin, which has been confirmed in meta-analysis of trials with all statins.

An alternative approach if the patient fails to reach target is the addition of ezetimibe, which has a mode of action that is complemen-tary to statins. It has been shown to lead to substantial reductions in cholesterol when added to statins in patients with diabetes. To date several double-blind, randomized endpoint trials with ezetimibe have been negative. However, a trial in patients with chronic kidney disease, one quarter of whom had diabetes, demonstrated reduc-tions in major vascular events, and a trial in patients following acute coronary syndromes is in progress.

A recent meta-analysis has demonstrated that fibrates as a class reduce cardiovascular outcomes. Subgroup analysis for coronary events showed no significant benefit in patients with diabetes. Fenofibrate is the fibrate that has been used in the majority of stud-ies in people with diabetes. It has not shown any clear reduction in cardiovascular events, either when used alone or in combination with a statin, but demonstrated reductions in the progression of diabetic retinopathy that require further evaluation.

5.4 Management of hypertension to reduce cardiovascular risk

5.4.1 Early studies in isolated systolic hypertension

The first clear evidence that blood pressure lowering was of ben-efit in people with diabetes was from studies in older patients with isolated systolic hypertension. Chlortalidone and nitrendipine (not licensed in the UK) reduced events in people with diabetes com-pared with placebo, with significant reductions in cardiovascular events, cardiovascular mortality, and all-cause mortality.

5.4.2 **UKPDS blood pressure study**

During recruitment to the UKPDS the high prevalence of hypertension was noted, so a blood pressure study was nested within the main study, comparing tight blood pressure control (mean blood pressure 144/82 mmHg) with less tight control (mean 154/87 mmHg). One-quarter of the total study population was also in the blood pressure study. Tight control was obtained with a blood pressure lowering regimen based on either captopril or atenolol, but many patients required three or more drugs.

Tight blood pressure control reduced both microvascular and macrovascular complications of diabetes. No differences were observed comparing treatment based on captopril, with treatment based on atenolol, but the study was statistically underpowered for this comparison.

5.4.3 **Blood pressure targets in diabetes**

The Hypertension Optimal Treatment (HOT) trial was a shorter study that aimed to compared the benefits of three diastolic blood pressure targets, <90, <85, and <80 mmHg, on major cardiovascular events. The separation between the groups was less than intended, and the achieved blood pressures were 144/85, 141/83 and 140/81 mmHg.

In the study overall there was a reduction in major cardiovascular events comparing the group that had a target of <85 mmHg compared to a target of <90 mmHg, but there was no further benefit with a lower target of <80 mmHg. Post hoc subgroup analysis of the 1501 diabetic subjects (8%) showed a further significant reduction in major cardiovascular events in diabetic patients allocated to the lower target blood pressure.

The ADVANCE trial included a blood pressure lowering study comparing a fixed combination of perindopril plus indapamide with placebo and demonstrated that blood pressure lowering to even lower levels (135/75 mmHg), and in patients not deemed to have hypertension at baseline, further reduced cardiovascular events in diabetic patients (Figure 5.4).

The ACCORD study included a blood pressure arm comparing standard therapy, targeting a systolic blood pressure <140 mmHg, and intensive therapy, targeting a systolic blood pressure <120 mmHg. There was no effect on the primary composite outcome of nonfatal myocardial infarction, nonfatal stroke or death from cardiovascular causes. A slight reduction was seen in strokes.

When taken together these studies indicate that tight control of blood pressure reduces events more than less tight control, and indicate that a target blood pressure of <130/80 mmHg is supported by evidence, but that several agents may be required to reach the target.

5.4.4 **Which anti-hypertensive drugs to use?**

The major benefit is the amount of blood pressure reduction, and many people with diabetes will require multiple agents to reach

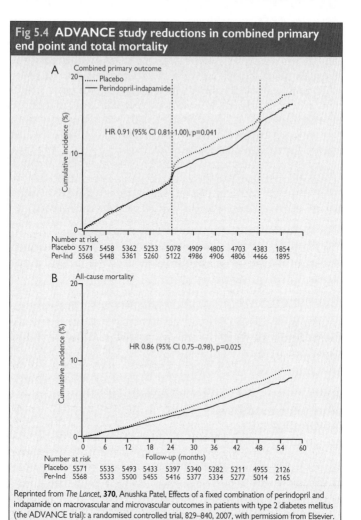

Fig 5.4 ADVANCE study reductions in combined primary end point and total mortality

A Combined primary outcome

HR 0.91 (95% CI 0.81–1.00), p=0.041

Number at risk
Placebo	5571	5458	5362	5253	5078	4909	4805	4703	4383	1854
Per-Ind	5568	5448	5361	5260	5122	4986	4906	4806	4466	1895

B All-cause mortality

HR 0.86 (95% CI 0.75–0.98), p=0.025

Follow-up (months)

Number at risk
Placebo	5571	5535	5493	5433	5397	5340	5282	5211	4955	2126
Per-Ind	5568	5533	5500	5455	5416	5377	5334	5277	5014	2165

Reprinted from The Lancet, **370**, Anushka Patel, Effects of a fixed combination of perindopril and indapamide on macrovascular and microvascular outcomes in patients with type 2 diabetes mellitus (the ADVANCE trial): a randomised controlled trial, 829–840, 2007, with permissiom from Elsevier.

blood pressure targets, so the question is not 'which drug to use?' but 'which drugs to use, and in what combinations?'. ACE inhibitors, angiotensin II receptor antagonists, calcium-channel blockers, beta-blockers, and diuretics are all proven to reduce events in people with diabetes. Recent studies have indicated that atenolol is less effective than other therapies in reducing blood pressure in people with diabetes, with a lesser reduction in cardiovascular events. First-line therapy is usually based on either an ACE inhibitor or angio-tensin II receptor antagonist, with subsequent addition of either a calcium-channel blocker or a diuretic (Figure 5.5).

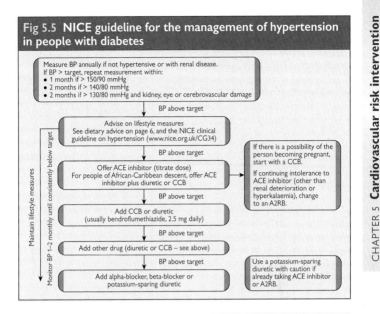

Fig 5.5 NICE guideline for the management of hypertension in people with diabetes

Measure BP annually if not hypertensive or with renal disease.
If BP > target, repeat measurement within:
• 1 month if > 150/90 mmHg
• 2 months if > 140/80 mmHg
• 2 months if > 130/80 mmHg and kidney, eye or cerebrovascular damage

↓ BP above target

Advise on lifestyle measures
See dietary advice on page 6, and the NICE clinical
guideline on hypertension (www.nice.org.uk/CG34)

↓ BP above target

Offer ACE inhibitor (titrate dose)
For people of African-Caribbean descent, offer ACE
inhibitor plus diuretic or CCB

If there is a possibility of the person becoming pregnant, start with a CCB.

If continuing intolerance to ACE inhibitor (other than renal deterioration or hyperkalaemia), change to an A2RB.

↓ BP above target

Add CCB or diuretic
(usually bendroflumethiazide, 2.5 mg daily)

↓ BP above target

Add other drug (diuretic or CCB – see above)

↓ BP above target

Add alpha-blocker, beta-blocker or
potassium-sparing diuretic

Use a potassium-sparing diuretic with caution if already taking ACE inhibitor or A2RB.

(left margin labels: Maintain lifestyle measures; Monitor BP 1–2 monthly until consistently below target)

5.5 Other approaches to cardiovascular risk reduction in diabetes

5.5.1 Multifactorial risk factor intervention

The Steno-2 study was a comparison of targeted, intensified, multi-factorial intervention with conventional treatment in a small group of patients with type 2 diabetes and microalbuminuria. Interventions in the intensive therapy group comprised advice on diet, exercise, and smoking cessation, intensive blood glucose control with a target HbA_{1c} below 6.5%, the use of an ACE inhibitor irrespective of blood pressure, aggressive treatment of hypertension, statins for raised cholesterol and fibrates for raised triglycerides, aspirin, and vitamin and mineral supplementation.

More patients in the intensive group reached targets for blood pressure, lipids and HbA_{1c}, and the HbA_{1c} targets were the hardest to achieve. Patients receiving intensive therapy had a significantly lower risk of cardiovascular disease, nephropathy, retinopathy, and autonomic neuropathy, with a 50% reduction in events over 8 years. Post trial monitoring out to 13 years showed a reduction in total and cardiovascular mortality.

5.5.2 Antiplatelet therapy

Aspirin was widely used in the past to reduce cardiovascular events in people with diabetes, but there is little evidence to support this.

A meta-analysis of antiplatelet therapy, mostly aspirin, showed a significant reduction in vascular events (non-fatal myocardial infarction, non-fatal stroke or vascular death) in diabetic patients with vascular disease.

Several recent meta-analyses of diabetic patients whose sole vascular risk factor was diabetes (i.e. primary prevention) showed no evidence of benefit from antiplatelet therapy, but clear evidence of harm with gastrointestinal bleeding and an increase in haemorrhagic strokes. Aspirin is no longer recommended for primary prevention of vascular events in people with diabetes.

5.5.3 **Antioxidants**

In the Steno-2 study a multivitamin preparation was included as antioxidant treatment. Many large, multicentre studies, including large numbers of patients with type 2 diabetes, have examined the possible reduction in cardiac events with antioxidant therapy, and these have been negative. A large study examining the possible benefits of aspirin and/or multivitamins in patients with type 2 diabetes is currently being run in the UK.

5.6 **Conclusions**

Multiple cardiovascular risk reduction is required in patients with type 2 diabetes, based on the use of statins to reduce cholesterol, multiple agents to reduce blood pressure, and the appropriate choice of antidiabetic drugs to control hyperglycaemia. The effects of aspirin are not proven in diabetic patients in the absence of vascular disease, and its use should be confined to patients with known cardiovascular disease.

References

Action to Control Cardiovascular Risk in Diabetes Study Group (2008) Effects of intensive glucose lowering in type 2 diabetes. *New England Journal of Medicine* **358**: 2545–59.

ADVANCE Collaborative Group (2007) Effects of a fixed combination of perindopril and indapamide on macrovascular and microvascular outcomes in patients with type 2 diabetes mellitus (the ADVANCE trial): a randomised controlled trial. *Lancet* **370**: 829–40.

ADVANCE Collaborative Group (2008) Intensive blood glucose control and vascular outcomes in patients with type 2 diabetes. *New England Journal of Medicine* **358**: 2560–72.

Antithrombotic Trialists' Collaboration (2002) Collaborative meta-analysis of randomised trials of antiplatelet therapy for prevention of death, myocardial infarction and stroke in high risk patients. *British Medical Journal* **324**: 71–86.

Cholesterol Treatment Trialists' (CTT) Collaborators (2008) Efficacy of cholesterol-lowering therapy in 18 686 people with diabetes in 14 randomised trials of statins: a meta-analysis. *Lancet* **371**: 117–25.

Dormandy, JA, Charbonnel, B, Eckland, DJ, *et al.* on behalf of the PROactive investigators (2005) Secondary prevention of macrovascular events in patients with type 2 diabetes in the PROactive study (PROspective pioglitAzone Clinical Trial in macroVascular Events): a randomised controlled trial. *Lancet* **366**: 1279–89.

Gaede P, Lund-Andersen H, Parving H-H, Pedersen O (2008) Effect of a multifactorial intervention on mortality in type 2 diabetes. *New England Journal of Medicine* **358**: 580–91.

Hansson, L, Zanchetti, A, Carruthers SG, *et al.* (1998) Effects of intensive blood-pressure lowering and low-dose aspirin in patients with hypertension: principal results of the Hypertension Optimal Treatment (HOT) randomised trial. *Lancet* **351**: 1755–62.

Holman RR, Paul SK, Bethel MA, Mathews DR, Neil HAW (2008) 10-year follow-up of intensive blood glucose control in type 2 diabetes. *New England Journal of Medicine* **359**: 1577–89.

Nissen SE, Wolski K (2007) Effect of rosiglitazone on the risk of myocardial infarction and death from cardiovascular causes. *New England Journal of Medicine* **356**: 2457–71.

Nissen SE, Wolski K (2010) Rosiglitazone revisited: an updated meta-analysis for risk of myocardial infarction and cardiovascular mortality. *Archives of Internal Medicine* **170**: 1191–201.

Ray KK, Seshasai SRK, Wijesuriya S, *et al.* (2009) Effect of intensive control of glucose on cardiovascular outcomes and death in patients with diabetes mellitus: a meta-analysis of randomised controlled trials. *Lancet* **373**: 1765–72.

Turner RC, Millns H, Neil HAW, *et al.* for the United Kingdom Prospective Diabetes Study Group. (1998). Risk factors for coronary artery disease in non-insulin dependent diabetes mellitus: United Kingdom prospective diabetes study (UPKDS: 23). *British Medical Journal*: **316**: 823–8.

UK Prospective Diabetes Study Group (1988) Tight blood pressure control and risk of macrovascular and microvascular complications in type 2 diabetes: UKPDS 38. *British Medical Journal*: **317**: 703–13.

UK Prospective Diabetes Study (UKPDS) Group (1998) Intensive blood-glucose control with sulphonylureas or insulin compared with conventional treatment and risk of complications in patients with type 2 diabetes (UKPDS 33). *Lancet* **352**: 837–53.

UK Prospective Diabetes Study (UKPDS) Group (1998) Effect of intensive blood glucose control with metformin on complications in overweight patients with type 2 diabetes (UKPDS 34). *Lancet* **352**: 854–65.

Chapter 6

Diet, exercise and other lifestyle factors

Katarina Kos and John PH Wilding

Key points

- All patients with type 2 diabetes, irrespective of their weight, should be advised to follow a healthy diet and be as physically active as possible
- Weight control is an essential part of the management of overweight and obese patients with type 2 diabetes; this may improve glucose metabolism and other risk factors
- Desirable lifestyle changes are alterations of the diet to one with a reduced energy intake and an increase in physical activity. Adherence to these changes requires behaviour modification and sustained motivation, so a multicomponent approach is recommended
- Anti-obesity drug therapy can help support lifestyle intervention, but should only be continued long term in patients who show clinical benefit
- Bariatric surgery, particularly gastric bypass, is highly effective in severely obese patients, providing remission of diabetes in about two-thirds of patients
- Other lifestyle recommendations—including smoking cessation, moderation of alcohol intake and salt reduction (in those with hypertension)—may be important for some patients.

6.1 Introduction

The average body mass index (BMI) at diagnosis of type 2 diabetes mellitus (T2DM) is typically at the high end of the overweight range, between 29 and 30 kg/m^2. Whilst the exact mechanisms through which obesity leads to T2DM remain incompletely understood, it is clear that an increased fat mass, especially intra-abdominal fat accumulation results in the metabolic syndrome which includes insulin resistance, hypertension and dyslipidaemia.

The presence of obesity (as assessed by an increased waist circumference) is considered an essential component of the metabolic syndrome using the latest International Diabetes Foundation (IDF) definition (2006). There is a very powerful relationship between being overweight or obese and the risk of developing T2DM, with a three-fold risk at a BMI of 25 kg/m^2, a 10-fold risk at a BMI of 30 kg/m^2, and a greater than 40-fold risk above a BMI of 35 kg/m^2 (Colditz et al., 1995), compared to a BMI of 22 kg/m^2. Due to an increasingly sedentary lifestyle and easy availability of energy-dense food, members of our society are becoming increasingly heavier by an estimated increase of 0.35 kg/year in body weight. More than 60% of the UK population is now overweight and 24% is obese. The excess weight consists primarily of fat tissue and is a result of positive energy balance in which energy intake is not offset by energy expenditure. Due to the increased risk of T2DM with obesity, the obesity epidemic is closely associated with a rapid increase in the incidence of type 2 diabetes. On the other hand, weight loss improves insulin resistance, and in subjects with impaired glucose tolerance, a 4% loss of body weight can reduce the risk of diabetes developing by 58% or more. There is also evidence that weight loss lowers blood pressure, improves lipid profiles and reduces HbA$_{1c}$ in people with diabetes (Look AHEAD Research Group, 2007) (Table 6.1). Thus, measures to slow the obesity epidemic are of paramount importance, and it is

Table 6.1 Benefits of 8% weight loss within 1 year in subjects with type 2 diabetes*	
Diabetes	10% decrease in fasting glucose Decrease in HbA$_{1c}$ by ≥0.5% 10% reduction in use of diabetes medication
Blood pressure	7 mmHg decrease in systolic pressure 3 mmHg decrease in diastolic pressure
Lipids	8% increase in HDL cholesterol 15% decrease in triglyceride levels 12% fewer lipid-lowering drug treatments from baseline in comparison to the control group
Albumin:creatinine ratio	Rate of normalization increased by 15%

* Comparison of intensive treatment in which lifestyle intervention, behaviour therapy and weight-reducing medication were compared with standard education in matched subjects with type 2 diabetes.

HDL, high density lipoprotein.

Data derived from the Look AHEAD Trial, 2007.

not surprising that obesity has moved up the political agenda, shown in the UK by the Foresight Report, *Tackling Obesities: Future Choices* (Government Office for Science, 2007).

6.2 **Lifestyle changes**

Modern society promotes a sedentary lifestyle, and an energy-dense, high fat diet makes it a challenge for individuals to maintain a healthy weight even in childhood, especially for those with a genetic predisposition to gain weight. This is exacerbated in a social environment where obesity is highly prevalent and likely to coexist in the whole family. Typically, weight gain develops gradually, nurtured by long-standing habits. Thus, it cannot be expected that a single educational session will solve this problem and change individuals' lifestyles to a degree by which they will stand out from a crowd in which obesogenic behaviour is the norm. Additionally, it has been shown that the expectations of obese patients with regards to weight loss become increasingly unrealistic as they become more obese. Failure to achieve their expectations results in frustration, which is frequently combined with low mood and sometimes clinical depressive illness. Long-term follow-up and continuous motivation for behaviour modification with avoidance of inconsistent messages from the healthcare team and avoidance of negative attitudes toward their problem are essential to aid weight management.

6.2.1 **Diet**

A diet that can be safely recommended for all patients with diabetes is a healthy balanced diet, low in fat and refined carbohydrate, combined with an energy reduction of 500–600 kcal/day from previous intake for patients who are overweight or obese (Broom, 2004) (Table 6.2). The recommended calorie intake can be calculated from age, gender and weight multiplied by a factor for activity, from several well-validated equations, and may be *greater* than

Table 6.2 Dietary recommendations for type 2 diabetes patients	
Carbohydrate	>55% of total energy Mostly of low glycaemic index
Fat Of which saturated fat	<35% of total energy <10% of total energy
Protein	10–15% of total energy
Fibre	>30g per day
Adapted from Broom (2004).	

the reported intake. In a diabetic patient, a modest weight loss of 5–10% can improve glycaemia as well as lipids and hypertension (see Table 6.1). Retrospective studies suggest that each kilogram of weight loss at 12 months after diagnosis of T2DM is associated with an increased survival of 3–4 months, which is more than can be achieved with glucose, lipid or blood pressure lowering alone. As such, advice to follow a sugar-free diet in itself is not sufficient—it is important to provide a clear and realistic target for weight loss from the onset.

It is known that obese subjects tend to underreport energy intake and that diabetic patients have more difficulties losing weight than non-diabetic individuals. This is partially due to the effects of some oral hypoglycaemic drugs (sulfonylureas and thiazolidinediones) and insulin in promoting weight gain. Education of patients and their understanding of the role of their diet and weight loss as part of the overall management plan to improve blood glucose are crucial. Patients should be advised to read food labels and encouraged to prepare their own meals whenever practical. Realistic goal setting facilitates continuous motivation and positive encouragement to avoid frustration (see Section 6.2.4).

Once the target has been reached, maintaining weight loss is perhaps the greatest challenge facing individuals. Even in intensive programmes, where intervention continues after weight loss has been achieved, such as in the Look Ahead study, there is often some weight regain, which leads to attenuation of the metabolic benefits. Although there are few long-term RCTs specifically addressing weight maintenance, data from the National Weight Control Registry from the USA suggests that people who successfully maintain weight loss regularly eat breakfast, keep to a healthy diet, undertake frequent self-monitoring of their weight, and undertake regular moderate physical activity for 30–60 minutes on most days.

6.2.2 Dietary approaches

In addition to the recommended low fat, moderately energy restricted diet discussed above, many other dietary approaches and terms are in common use. It should be noted that these dietary approaches are not all mutually exclusive. They are briefly described below.

6.2.2.1 Low calorie diets (LCDs)

By definition these diets should provide a sustainable reduction in energy intake that is below requirements, e.g. to an approximate energy intake of 1000–1600 kcal/day. A 500–1000 kcal deficit per day will lead to an approximate weight loss of 0.5–1.0 kg per week.

6.2.2.2 Very low calorie diets (VLCDs)

These are usually diets providing <600 kcal/day and are marketed as a total food substitute (e.g. Slim-Fast®). VLCDs should only be used under dietetic and medical supervision for short-term periods, but may be of benefit to patients who are unable to lose weight using other approaches. Long-term use of the VLCD approach in diabetes does not have an improved sustained weight benefit in comparison to standard approaches (Paisey et al., 2002).

6.2.2.3 Low fat diets (LFDs)

A reduction in total fat intake is the easiest way to reduce total energy intake. The estimated energy intake on LFDs is usually >1600 kcal/day and, with a high proportion of essential fatty acids, considered nutritionally the safest. Data from a systematic review of randomized controlled trials of the long-term benefits of weight-reducing diets in adults supports the use of LFDs for weight reduction.

6.2.2.4 Low glycaemic index (GI) diets

In this approach, patients are advised to avoid unrefined sugars and base carbohydrate intake on complex carbohydrates with a low GI index, e.g. wholemeal breads, porridge, pasta and beans. An improvement in blood glucose can be achieved by long-term adherence (Rizkalla et al., 2004).

6.2.2.5 Low carbohydrate diets

The best known low carbohydrate diet is carbohydrate substitution by high protein content, e.g. the Atkins diet or the protein-sparing modified fast (PSMF) diet. It is suggested that these diets promote ketone production, which suppresses appetite. However, these diets tend to be high in fat, remain controversial, and are not routinely recommended in people with diabetes. Some recent research suggests that recommending a diet that is both high in protein (aiming for 25% of energy) and of low glycaemic index may be better for weight maintenance than other approaches, but this has not yet been tested in people with diabetes (Larsen et al., 2010).

6.2.2.6 Meal replacements

These are commercially available low energy foods, which are either based on a low carbohydrate content of <40 g/day (e.g. Optifast®, Modifast®) or are nutrient complete, low energy diets (e.g. Slim-Fast®, see Section 6.2.2.2). There is some evidence that this approach may be of benefit in some patients with diabetes in the short term, but long-term data are lacking.

Whilst initiation of diet has been regarded as first-line treatment of diabetes before the initiation of drug therapy, withholding antidiabetic drug therapy is not justified if the blood glucose is high. According to the UK Prospective Diabetes Study (UKPDS) 7 (UKPDS Group, 1990), an average weight loss of 16% would be needed to normalize the fasting blood sugar from an initial 6–8 mmol/L to less than 6 mmol/L. This is a far greater weight loss than can be achieved by most patients for remission of their diabetes. However, diet remains one of the most important components of successful

T2DM therapy, and a short term (three months) trial of diet and life-style with the aim of weight loss is a reasonable first step of management in newly diagnosed patients without severe hyperglycaemia (NICE 2009).

6.2.3 **Exercise**

There are numerous molecular explanations of how exercise improves insulin sensitivity, whilst a causality of diabetes as consequence of lack of exercise is not proven. Exercise substantially decreases the risk of T2DM and improves blood glucose control irrespective of the weight effect of physical activity. Whilst physical activity alone is less effective than dietary treatment for weight loss itself, exercise reduces abdominal fat and prevents further weight gain. People who exercise the most are the least likely to be obese, and gain less weight with age. There has been recent interest in the relative benefits of aerobic vs resistance exercise in helping blood glucose control in diabetes. In reality, a mixture of both is probably optimal. For people who have type 2 diabetes, the latest guidelines recommend at least 150 minutes per week of moderate to vigorous aerobic exercise spread out at least 3 days during the week, with no more than 2 consecutive days between bouts of aerobic activity, plus resistance exercise at least 2 days per week. In obese individuals who have lost weight, a higher level of activity (30–60 minutes per day on most days of the week), may be necessary to help maintain weight. Whatever exercise is chosen, activity levels need to be built up slowly with consideration of the individual's fitness and co-morbidities. Examples of adequate physical activities are listed in Table 6.3.

These levels of activity are equivalent to using 150–200 kcal, depending on the patient's weight and the level of activity. It is

Table 6.3 Examples of moderate amounts of physical activity	
Common chores	**Sporting activities**
Gardening for 30–45 minutes	Walking 2.8 km (1.75 miles) in 35 minutes (20 min/mile)
Raking leaves for 30 minutes	Running 2.4 km (1.5 miles) in 15 minutes (10 minutes/mile)
Washing and waxing a car for 45–60 minutes	Swimming for 20 minutes
Washing windows or floors for 45–60 minutes	Cycling 8 km (5 miles) in 30 minutes
Stair-walking for 15 minutes	Dancing fast (social) for 30 minutes
Adapted from NIH (2000).	

important to carefully evaluate patients with type 2 diabetes prior to them embarking on an exercise programme, especially if they are at high risk of cardiovascular disease; patients with a previous cardiac history, autonomic neuropathy or long duration of diabetes may require formal evaluation. Patients with significant proliferative retinopathy should also avoid high intensity exercise until this has been adequately treated (ADA guidelines, 2010).

6.2.4 **Behaviour modification**

Cognitive behaviour therapy clearly has its benefits in the achievement of sustained weight loss, and its addition to diet and exercise is valuable. The approach does not differ from the one recommended for non-diabetic patients. However, due to resource issues behaviour modification elements should be integrated in primary care visits as well as diabetes clinics and be incorporated in all consultations. Behaviour therapy is aimed at controlling signals and behaviour that lead to obesity, but also for the patient to learn to deal with lapses. Core elements of behaviour therapies are to involve the patient through an increase in motivation and realistic expectations and target setting (e.g. loss of 5–10% of body weight in 6 months with reasonable short-term goals of 0.5–1 kg/week). A progress review at reasonable time intervals appears beneficial.

The ideal body weight is usually not an achievable target and should not be aimed for. Generally, it is inappropriate to institute negative attitudes to the patient's old dietary habits and lifestyle, but to work by positive reinforcement and aim at slow attitude changes and small sustainable weight losses (Jebb et al., 2003).

6.2.5 **Synergistic effect of therapies**

The combination of behaviour therapy, exercise and diet is more effective than any one alone and they are therefore used in combination (Table 6.4). A recent Cochrane review suggested that a 1% reduction of HbA_{1c} could be achieved after 12 months of diet and exercise. Lifestyle changes should thus be continued and maintained throughout the addition of any other interventions (Nield et al., 2007).

6.2.6 **Pharmacotherapy for weight loss**

The only currently licensed drug suitable for weight management in diabetes is the intestinal lipase inhibitor orlistat. Orlistat can be used in patients with T2DM with a BMI of >28 kg/m^2 (Torgerson, 2004) (NICE, 2006; Padwal & Majumdar, 2007); its effects are modest, with an additional 2.7 kg weight loss when used in combination with a lifestyle support programme in patients with T2DM (NICE, 2006). Because of its mode of action, orlistat may cause fatty stools leading to diarrhoea, and is not always well tolerated by patients, particularly if the diet remains high in fat. The licensing requirements of orlistat require an initial weight loss of 5% from baseline after

Table 6.4 Key characteristics of successful dietary weight control (adapted from Jebb, 2003)

• Regular weighing
• Regular meals and snacks
• Smaller portion sizes
• Restricted intake of energy-dense foods
• Reduced fat and fat cooking methods
• Proportionally more carbohydrates of low glycaemic index
• Increased fruit and vegetable intake
• Increased physical activity
• Small, realistic goals setting
• Support from family and friends

3 months treatment to continue treatment beyond this time, and the drug should be stopped if significant weight regain occurs. Whilst drug therapies have their role in supporting weight control, like any other drug for chronic disease management, their weight-reducing effect is usually not sustained once the drug is withdrawn, so long-term treatment is likely to be necessary for weight maintenance. However, considering the natural tendency of weight increase, maintenance of body weight may be considered a success.

6.2.7 **Bariatric surgery**

Bariatric surgery (surgery that aids weight reduction) is currently recommended by the National Institute for Health and Clinical Excellence (NICE, 2006) for patients with a BMI of >40 kg/m² or >35 kg/m² with co-morbidities such as diabetes. These procedures do not only lead to effective weight loss, but improve insulin sensitivity, and, in the most recent analyses, reduce mortality from vascular disease and cancer in the long term (Sjöström et al., 2007). Whilst the most popular procedure is gastric banding, gastric bypass leads to a greater improvement and, in about two-thirds of cases, remission of diabetes which could be at least partially related to a favourable change of gut hormones that regulate insulin secretion and appetite. These therapies require long-term follow-up, and despite NICE recommendations these interventions are yet to achieve widespread acceptance in the UK.

6.2.8 **Others**

Apart from lifestyle changes with the aim of weight maintenance or reduction, there are other important measures aimed at cardiovascular risk reduction. Smoking cessation can be aided by smoking cessation programs and the use of nicotine replacement therapy or drugs. In addition, subjects with raised blood pressure should be recommended to restrict their salt intake. A reduction of alcohol intake will aid overall calorie restriction, but reduce the risk of hypoglycaemia, particularly in patients treated with insulin and/or sulfonylureas.

References

American Diabetes Association (2010) Exercise and type 2 Diabetes. Position Statement. *Diabetes Care* **33**: 2692.

Broom I (2004) Diet and food-based therapies for obesity in diabetic patients. In: AH Barnett, S Kumar (eds) *Obesity and Diabetes*. John Wiley & Sons Ltd, Chichester.

Colditz GA, Willett WC, Rotnitzky A, Manson JE (1995) Weight gain as a risk factor for clinical diabetes in women. *Ann Intern Med* **121**: 481–6.

Government Office for Science (2007) Foresight Report. Tackling Obesities: Future Choices. Project Report. www.foresight.gov.uk/Obesity/obesity_final/17.pdf.

IDF (International Dibetes Foundation) (2006) IDF Consensus World wide Definition of the Metabolic Syndrome www.idf.org/webdata/docs/IDF_Meta_def_final.pdf.

Jebb SA, Steer T (2003) *Tackling the Weight of the Nation*. MRC, Cambridge.

Kos K, Baker C, Kumar S (2005) Current treatment strategies for obesity. *Therapy* **6**: 955–67.

Larsen TM, Dalskov MS, van Baak M, *et al.* for the Diet, Obesity, and Genes (Diogenes) Project (2010) Diets with High or Low Protein Content and Glycemic Index for Weight-Loss Maintenance. *N Engl J Med* **363**; 2102–13.

Look AHEAD Research Group, Pi-Sunyer X, Blackburn G, Brancati FL, *et al.* (2007) Reduction in weight and cardiovascular disease risk factors in individuals with type 2 diabetes: one-year results of the Look AHEAD trial. *Diabet Care* **30**: 1374–83.

Look AHEAD Research Group (2010) Long-term effects of a lifestyle intervention on weight and cardiovascular risk factors in individuals with type 2 diabetes mellitus: four-year results of the Look AHEAD trial. *Archives of Internal Medicine* **70**: 1566–75.

NICE (National Institute for Health and Clinical Excellence) (2006) Obesity Guidance on the Prevention, Identification, Assessment and Management of Overweight and Obesity in Adults and Children. www.nice.org.uk/nicemedia/pdf/word/CG43NICEGuideline.doc.65.

NIH (National Institutes of Health) (2000) The Practical Guide: Identification, Evaluation, and Treatment of Overweight and Obesity in Adults. www.nhlbi.nih.gov/guidelines/obesity/practgde.htm.

Nield L, Moore HJ, Hooper L, *et al.* (2007) Dietary advice for treatment of type 2 diabetes mellitus in adults (review). *Cochrane Database of Systematic Reviews*. John Wiley & Sons Ltd, Chichester.

Padwal RS, Majumdar SR (2007) Drug treatments for obesity: orlistat, sibutramine, and rimonabant. *Lancet* **369**: 71–7.

Paisey RB, Frost J, Harvey P, *et al.* (2002) Five year results of a prospective very low calorie diet or conventional weight loss programme in type 2 diabetes. *J Hum Nutr Diet* **15**: 121–7.

Rizkalla SW, Taghrid L, Laromiguiere M, *et al.* (2004) Improved plasma glucose control, whole-body glucose utilization, and lipid profile on a low-glycemic index diet in type 2 diabetic men: a randomized controlled trial. *Diabet Care* **27**: 1866–72.

Rössner S, Sjöström L, Noack R, *et al.* (2000) Weight loss, weight maintenance, and improved cardiovascular risk factors after 2 years treatment with orlistat for obesity. European Orlistat Obesity Study Group. *Obes Res* **8**: 49–61.

Sjöström L, Narbro K, Sjöström CD, *et al.* (2007) Swedish obese subjects study, effects of bariatric surgery on mortality in Swedish obese subjects. *N Engl J Med* **357**: 741–52.

Torgerson JS, Hauptman J, Boldrin MN, Sjostrom L (2004) XENical in the prevention of Diabetes in Obese Subjects (XENDOS) study: a randomized study of orlistat as an adjunct to lifestyle changes for the prevention of type 2 diabetes in obese patients. *Diabet Care* **27**: 155–61.

UKPDS (UK Prospective Diabetes Study) Group (1990) Response of fasting plasma glucose to diet therapy in newly presenting type 2 diabetic patients (UKPDS 7). *Metabolism* **39**: 905–12.

Chapter 7

Managing glycaemia—current oral agents

Roger Gadsby

> **Key points**
> - Once treatment with lifestyle modification fails to achieve optimal control of glycaemia, oral glucose lowering agents are required. Initially one oral agent is used in monotherapy
> - If treatment with one agent doesn't achieve optimal glycaemic control a second oral agent can be added in dual therapy
> - If two agents are not successful, a third can be added, in triple oral therapy
> - Such combination therapy is possible as there are different groups of agents that lower blood glucose by different mechanisms.

7.1 Glucose lowering efficacy of oral agents

A systematic review (Bolen *et al.*, 2007) of 216 trials and cohort studies and two systematic reviews concluded that glitazones and metformin lower HbA_{1c} to the same degree as sulfonylureas (about a 1–1.5% reduction depending on starting HbA_{1c}).

The choice of which oral glucose-lowering agent to use has therefore to be made on other considerations, apart from glucose-lowering efficacy (see Table 7.1). There is however a difference in their speed of action. Sulfonylureas work within a few days, metformin takes a few weeks, and glitazones can take up to 6 months to achieve their maximal drop in HbA_{1c}.

7.2 Biguanide—Metformin

Metformin is the only agent in the biguanide class available in the UK and has been marketed for 50 years. Its main side effects are on the gastrointestinal tract where it can cause abdominal pain, nausea, diarrhoea and a metallic taste in the mouth. Around 10–20% of patients do not continue on generic metformin because of these side effects. They can be minimized by starting with a low dose, say 500 mg daily and titrating up to 500 mg three times daily over 2 to 4 weeks.

Metformin is excreted in the urine. A rare serious side effect associated with metformin is lactic acidosis, and this may be more likely to happen if metformin accumulates in the body when there is renal impairment. Guidelines (NICE, 2008) therefore suggest stopping metformin if the serum creatinine level rises above 150 micromol/l or the eGFR is below 30 ml/minute/1.73m^2 and reviewing the dose of metformin if the serum creatinine exceeds 130 micromol/l or the eGFr is below 45 ml/minute/1.73m^2. Because of the increased risk of lactic acidosis metformin is contraindicated in people with uncontrolled heart failure and advanced liver disease. The UKPDS study demonstrated in a subgroup of overweight patients with newly diagnosed Type 2 diabetes that intensive glucose-lowering treatment with metformin was associated with a 32% risk reduction for diabetes-related endpoints (including MI and stroke) and a 42% reduction in risk for diabetes-related deaths compared with conventional treatment with diet alone (UK Prospective Diabetes Study (UKPDS) Group, 1998a). Metformin was the only glucose-lowering agent in the UKPDS study to improve cardiovascular outcomes in this group of patients. On the strength of these findings metformin is the unequivocal first-line pharmacological therapy of choice in the majority of patients with Type 2 diabetes and the foundation of oral glucose lowering treatment.

7.3 **Extended-absorption metformin**

A once-daily formulation of metformin has recently been released, and can be given as 1 to 4 tablets once a day. It is said to cause less diarrhoea and GI side effects than the generic preparation and should be considered where GI intolerability prevents continuation of metformin therapy (NICE, 2008).

Table 7.1 Classes of oral agents

Biguanide	Decreases hepatic gluconeogenesis and inceases peripheral glucose uptake
Sulfonylureas & prandial glucose regulators	Stimulate pancreatic *beta* cells to release insulin
Thiazolidinediones (glitazones)	Interact with PPARγ to upregulate transcription of insulin responsive genes
Alpha-glucosidase inhibitors	Delays absorption of glucose from gut

Table 7.2 Sulfonylureas available in the UK	
Glibenclamide	5–15 mg daily
Gliclazide	40–320 mg daily
Gliclazide MR	30–120 mg daily
Glimepiride	1–6 mg daily
Glipizide	2.5–20 mg daily
Tolbutamide	500 mg–2g daily

7.4 Sulfonylureas

There are 5 sulfonylureas available in the UK in July 2010 (see Table 7.2). The main difference between members of the group is duration of action. Hypoglycaemia is the main side effect. This is more likely to occur with glibenclamide, because of its long half-life.

Sulfonylureas also cause weight gain. They should be avoided in people with severe renal and liver impairment.

7.5 Prandial glucose regulators

The agents repaglinide and nateglinide are available in the UK. These short-acting insulin secretagogues work within 10–30 mins of ingestion and have a duration of action of 2 to 4 hours. They are therefore given with each meal. They work on the same receptor in the beta-cell as do sulfonylureas, and stimulate insulin release. Repaglinide can be used in monotherapy or with metformin. Nateglinide can only be used in combination with metformin. These short-acting agents are taken with each meal, so they are useful if people have erratic eating patterns, e.g. shift workers. As a result of this mode of action they have a similar potential to cause hypoglycaemia. They have not gained wide use.

7.6 Thiazolidinediones (glitazones)

Two thiazolidinediones or glitazones are available in the UK. They are pioglitazone and rosiglitazone. While the European Medicines Agency (EMA) has suspended authorization for rosiglitazone, another glitazone (pioglitazone) is still available in the UK and elsewhere. The main side effect is fluid retention with increased plasma volume, reduced haematocrit, and a decrease in haemoglobin. As a result peripheral oedema, mainly at the ankles, may occur in some patients. There may be an associated weight gain of around 5%. There is an increased risk of congestive cardiac failure but not of mortality from heart failure described in a recent systematic review and meta-analysis (Largo, 2007).

A previously released glitazone called troglitazone was withdrawn due to cases of fatal hepatotoxicity. Pioglitazone and rosiglitazone has been used extensively and none of the liver toxicity found with troglitazone has been reported. There is therefore no requirement for 2 monthly liver function test monitoring for glitazones.

Combination tablets of metformin and pioglitazone are now available in the UK. Glitazones have been shown to reduce blood pressure slightly, and pioglitazone will reduce total cholesterol by around 15%. It was hoped that these improvements in surrogate markers for cardiovascular disease (CVD) would result in reductions in CVD adverse outcomes. A very recent systematic review (Lincoff, 2007) of 19 trials has concluded that pioglitazone does reduce the rate of death, myocardial infarction and stroke by 18% compared with controls. However two similar meta-analyses for rosiglitazone (Nissen, 2007; Singh, 2007) suggest an increase in risk of myocardial infarction of around 40%.

Recently the EMA has studied concerns regarding a possible increased risk of bladder cancer with pioglitazone. They believe the risk may be real but have concluded that the benefits outweigh the risks in a limited number of patients. They request further work in this area by the licence holder. They caution against its use in patients at increased risk of bladder cancer (the elderly, cigarette smokers, those exposed to certain drugs and chemicals) and add that the drug is contraindicated in people with current or past bladder cancer or in those with uninvestigated haematuria.

7.7 Alpha-glucosidase inhibitors

The only agent that is available in the UK is acarbose. It can reduce HbA_{1c} between 0.6–1%, a slightly lower reduction than that from the 3 previous classes. Its mode of action to delay absorption of sugars in the small intestine means that the extra carbohydrate that gets into the large bowel is digested by bowel micro organisms producing flatulence, bloating and diarrhoea. These side effects mean that the agent is little used in the UK.

7.8 Using the current oral agents—in initial monotherapy

Metformin is the recommended oral agent for initial monotherapy in people with type 2 diabetes who are overweight in current national and international guidelines (NICE, 2009; IDF 2005; Nathan, 2006) The reasons for this include that it is well known, it is cheap, it doesn't cause hypoglycaemia, it is weight neutral, and it has been shown to reduce CVD risk in the UKPDS metformin substudy (UKPDS, 1998). It should also be considered as oral monotherapy in people who are of normal weight (NICE, 2009). The small group of patients who newly present with diabetes who are thin, who eat healthily and who have significant symptoms of hyperglycaemia such as thirst, polydypsia and polyuria are perhaps the only group who may be better treated by a sulfonylurea rather than metformin initially. The sulfonylurea will act more quickly to relieve symptoms and lack of insulin rather than insulin resistance might be felt to be the major problem in such individuals.

7.9 Using the current agents—dual therapy

Once treatment with lifestyle modification followed by metformin therapy is insufficient to optimize glycaemic control, the 2009 NICE guidelines (NICE, 2009) recommend the addition of sulfonylurea, as do the IDF guidelines (IDF, 2005). The reasons for this include the fact that the agents have been around for a long time and are well known, that they act quickly and effectively lower blood glucose, and that they are cheap. The IDF guidelines (IDF 2005) suggest that the addition of a glitazone to metformin for dual therapy could be an option. The ADA/EASD guideline (Nathan, 2006) suggests that after metformin, either a sulfonylurea, or a glitazone or insulin initiation might be considered as options for dual therapy. Glitazones have been promoted by their manufacturers for use as second to metformin on the basis that they lower HbA$_{1c}$ as well as sulfonylurea (although they take longer to do this), they do not cause hypoglycaemia and that they may well lower CVD risk. There is emerging evidence to support the lowering of CVD risk for pioglitazone (Lincoff, 2007; Tzoulaki, 2010). The evidence from meta-analysis for rosiglitazone suggests it does not decrease risk but may increase risk (Nissen, 2007; Singh, 2007; Tzoulaki, 2010). Pioglitazone came off patent in early 2011. It is likely that its cost will then drop considerably, although this is yet to be seen. Even with a reduction in cost, the recent safety concerns will influence whether this drug continues in common usage. However, if pioglitazone then costs around the same amount as a sulfonylurea the choice as to which generic therapy to use with metformin will become more difficult.

7.10 Triple therapy

Once metformin and sulfonylurea taken in dual therapy at maximally tolerated doses are not sufficient for optimal control of glycaemia, what options are available? At present in the UK the options are:

1 add a glitazone in a 'triple oral therapy' combination

2 add insulin

3 add an injectable GLP-1 agonist (exenatide and liraglutide are currently available)

4 add a DPP4 inhibitor (at present the only DPP4 inhibitor licensed for use in triple therapy is sitagliptin).

GLP-1 agonists and DPP4 inhibitors are discussed in another chapter, as are the details of the use of insulin, so only the use of a glitazone or insulin in general terms will be discussed here. Several studies have compared the option of insulin or glitazone in triple therapy (Alijabri, 2004; Rosenstock, 2006) They have shown similar levels of HbA$_{1c}$ in the group given glitazone in triple oral therapy and the group given basal insulin and dual oral therapy. Depending on how many units of insulin are required the costs of each option can be similar. In view of the data on glitazones and CVD risk discussed above, pioglitazone at a dose of 30mg once daily should be the preferred glitazone in the triple oral agent option. When given the choice a number of patients opt for triple oral therapy rather than 2 tablets and the injection of insulin.

Box 7.1 Costs of oral hypoglycaemic agents for 28 days treatment

Metformin 4 of 500 mg tabs/daily	£1.83
Metformin modified release 4 of 500 mg/daily	£12.28
Gliclazide 2 of 80 mg/daily	£1.51
Gliclazide modified release 2 of 30 mg/daily	£5.92
Pioglitazone 30 mg/daily	£33.25
Metformin/pioglitazone 2 of 850 mg/15 mg/daily	£31.56

Pioglitazone came off patent in early 2011 and its price is expected to drop towards the average generic price of £2–3 within the next 1–2 years. Modified from Prescribing for Diabetes in England—An update 2002–2008

Box 7.2 Items prescribed and dispensed in England

	Jan–March 2002	Jan–March 2004	Jan–March 2006	Jan–March 2008
Metformin	1.2 million	1.7 million	2.3 million	2.6 million
Sulfonylureas	1.2 million	1.2 million	1.2 million	1.5 million
Others	0.2 million	0.3 million	0.5 million	0.6 million

Approximate numbers modified from Prescribing for Diabetes in England—An update 2002–2008

Box 7.3 Approximate costs modified from Prescribing for Diabetes in England Nov 2007

	Jan–March 2002	Jan–March 2004	Jan–March 2006	Jan–March 2008
Metformin	£4 million	£5 million	£10 million	£9 million
Sulfonylureas	£9 million	£9 million	£8 million	£5 million
Others	£5 million	£12 million	£22 million	£26 million

Source: Prescribing for Diabetes in England—An update 2002-2008 published June 2009 by The NHS Information Centre and Yorkshire and Humberside Public Health Observatory, www.yhpho.org.uk.

References

Aljabri K, Kosak S, Thompson DM (2004) Addition of pioglitazone or bedtime insulin to maximal doses of sulphonylurea and metformin in type 2 diabetes patients with poor glucose control: a prospective randomized study. Am J Med **116**: 230–5.

Blonde L, Dailey GE, Jabbour SA, et al. (2004) Gastrointestinal tolerability of extended-release metformin compared to immediate release metformin tablets: results of a retrospective cohort study. Current Med Res and Opinions **20**: 565–72.

Bolen S, Feldman L, Vassey J, et al. (2007) Systematic review: comparative effectiveness and safety of oral medications for type 2 diabetes. Ann Int Med **147**: 386–99.

IDF (2005) Global guideline for type 2 diabetes. IDF, Brussels, www.idg.org.

Largo RM, Singh PP, Nesto RW (2007) Congestive cardiac failure and cardiovascular death in patients with pre-diabetes and type 2 diabetes given thiazolidinediones: a meta-analysis of randomized controlled trials. Lancet **370**: 1129–36.

Lincoff AM, Wolski K, Nicholls SJ, Nissen SJ (2007) Pioglitazone and risk of cardiovascular events in patients with type 2 diabetes: a meta-analysis of randomized controlled trials. JAMA **298**: 1180–8.

McGavin JK, Perry CM, Goa KL (2002) Gliclazide modified release. Drugs **62**: 1357–64.

Nathan DM, Buse JB, Davidson MB, et al. (2006) Management of hyperglycemia in type 2 diabetes: A consensus algorithm for the initiation and adjustment of therapy: a consensus statement from the American Diabetes Association and the European Association for the Study of Diabetes. Diabetes Care **29**: 1963–72.

NICE (2008) Type 2 diabetes: National Clinical Guideline for management in Primary & Secondary Care (CG66). NICE, London.

NICE (2009) Type 2 Diabetes: The management of type 2 diabetes (CG 87). NICE, London.

Nissen SE, Wolski K (2007) Effects of rosiglitazone on the risk of myocardial infarction and Death from cardiovasdcular causes. N Engl J Med **357**: 2457–71.

Rosenstock J, Sugimoto D, Strange P, *et al.* (2006) Triple therapy in type 2 diabetes. *Diabetes Care* **29**: 554–9.

Singh S, Loke YK, Furberg CD (2007) Long-term risk of cardiovascular events with rosiglitazone: a meta-analysis. *JAMA* **298**: 1189–95.

Tzoulaki I, Molokhia M, Curcin V, *et al.* (2010) Risk of cardiovascular disease and all cause mortality among patients with type 2 diabetes prescribed oral antidiabetic drugs: retrospective cohort study using UK general practice research database. *BMJ* **339**: b4731 Published 2 Jan 2010 vol. 340.

UK Prospective Diabetes Study (UKPDS) Group (1998a) Effect intensive blood glucose control with metformin on complications in overweight patients with type 2 diabetes (UKPDS 34). *Lancet* **352**: 854–65.

Chapter 8

Managing glycaemia: recently introduced and future therapies

Clifford J Bailey and Caroline Day

Key points

- Established blood glucose-lowering agents exert valuable effects in the management of type 2 diabetes, but they do not entirely normalize metabolic control: hence the need for additional therapies
- New formulations of some established agents and single tablet 'fixed-dose' combinations offer improved efficacy with reduced side effects, and assist in reducing 'pill burden'
- Glucagon-like peptide-1 (GLP-1) receptor agonists, namely exenatide and liraglutide, are subcutaneously injected peptide analogues of GLP-1 that increase prandial insulin secretion, reduce glucagon secretion and facilitate weight loss
- Inhibitors of the enzyme dipeptidyl peptidase-IV (DPP-4), known as gliptins (e.g. sitagliptin, vildagliptin and saxagliptin) are oral agents that prevent the degradation of endogenous GLP-1, providing a further means to enhance prandial insulin secretion
- The dopamine D_2 agonist bromocriptine, the bile sequestrant colesevelam, and the soluble amylin analogue pramlintide have received glucose-lowering indications in some countries outside of Europe
- Potential new types of blood glucose-lowering agents in development include inhibitors of the renal sodium-glucose cotransporter-2 (SGLT2), activators of the glucose-phosphorylating enzyme glucokinase, and inhibitors of the glucocorticoid-activating enzyme 11β-hydroxysteroid dehydrogenase-1 (11βHSD1).

8.1 **Abstract**

Several new and modified therapies have been introduced to improve the management of hyperglycaemia. To enhance tolerability, metformin is now available as a slow-release tablet, a liquid formulation and a powder sachet that dissolves in water. Various single tablet 'fixed-dose' combinations, mostly containing metformin with another oral antidiabetic agent can reduce the pill burden of type 2 diabetes. The incretin system has provided two new types of agents. Glucagon-like peptide-1 (GLP-1) receptor agonists (exenatide and liraglutide) are subcutaneously injected stable analogues of GLP-1 that reduce hyperglycaemia by increasing prandial insulin secretion and reducing glucagon secretion. These effects are glucose-dependent, minimizing the risk of hypoglycaemic episodes, and a mild satiety effect facilitates weight loss. To enhance the activity of endogenous GLP-1, which is normally degraded rapidly by the enzyme dipeptidyl peptidase-IV (DPP-4), several DPP-4 inhibitors (termed gliptins) have been developed (sitagliptin, vildagliptin, saxagliptin). These agents act mainly to reduce prandial glycaemia via enhanced glucose-dependent insulin responses that carry low risk of hypoglycaemia and do not cause weight gain. In some countries the dopamine agonist bromocriptine, the bile sequestrant colesevelam and the soluble amylin analogue pramlintide are approved as glucose-lowering agents. Inhibitors of the renal sodium-glucose cotransporter-2 (SGLT2) may provide a future non-insulin dependent method of lowering blood glucose by eliminating excess glucose into the urine.

8.2 **Introduction**

Despite an increasing variety of medications for the treatment of hyperglycaemia (Table 8.1), many diabetes patients do not achieve or sustain recommended glycaemic targets: micro- and macro-vascular complications are still rife, and the quality and quantity of life is seriously compromised.

For type 1 diabetes the life-preserving properties of insulin are crucial, but the ongoing challenge is to mimic physiological insulin delivery as closely as possible. With type 2 diabetes, the highly heterogeneous and progressive pathophysiology requires different agents to address different aspects of the disease at different stages of its natural history. Typically, insulin resistance and pancreatic beta-cell dysfunction are well established at the time of diagnosis, and continued deterioration of beta-cell function largely dictates further escalation of the hyperglycaemia. In consequence, the treatment algorithm customarily involves up-titration of glucose-lowering

Table 8.1 Classes of established and new antidiabetic drugs and their main mechanisms of action (based on Krentz & Bailey (2005) *Drugs* 65: 385–411)

Class	Examples[a]	Main mechanisms of action	Administration route
Insulins	*Rapid-acting:* aspart, lispro, glulisine. *Short-acting:* Actrapid®, Humulin S®, Insuman® Rapid *Intermediate:* Insulatard®, Humulin I® *Long-acting:* glargine, detemir *Biphasic:* Humulin M3®, Insuman Comb®	Reduce hepatic glucose output Increase peripheral glucose uptake Increase glucose metabolism Decrease lipolysis Increase lipogenesis Favour protein anabolism	SC injection[b]
Sulfonylureas	Glibenclamide[c], gliclazide, glimepiride, glipizide, tolbutamide	Stimulate insulin secretion (effect typically lasts 6–24 h)	Oral
Meglitinides (prandial insulin releasers, glinides)	Repaglinide, nateglinide	Stimulate insulin secretion (rapid effect, typically lasts <6 h)	Oral
Biguanide	Metformin	Improves insulin action and exerts some insulin-independent effects	Oral
Thiazolidinediones	Pioglitazone, rosiglitazone[e]	Improve insulin action mainly via PPARγ agonism	Oral
Alpha-glucosidase inhibitors	Acarbose, miglitol[d], voglibose[d]	Slow rate of carbohydrate digestion	Oral

(Continued)

CHAPTER 8 **Recent and future therapies**

Table 8.1 (*Contd'*)

Class	Examples[a]	Main mechanisms of action	Administration route
GLP-1[e] receptor agonists (GLP-1 analogues/mimetics)	Exenatide, liraglutide	Mimic GLP-1[e]: enhance prandial insulin secretion	SC injection[b]
DPP-4 inhibitors (gliptins)	Sitagliptin, vildagliptin, saxagliptin	Inhibit DPP-4[f]: enhance prandial insulin secretion	Oral
Amylin analogue	Pramlintide[d]	Suppress glucagon secretion and slow gastric emptying	SC injection[b]
Dopamine agonist	Bromocriptine	Improve circadian rhythmicity of glycaemic control	Oral
Bile sequestrant	Colesevelam	Possibly alter incretin secretions	Oral

[a]Availability of agents and prescribing instructions vary between countries.
[b]Administered by subcutaneous injection.
[c]Glibenclamide is called glyburide in some countries.
[d]Not available in UK.
[e]Glucagon-like peptide-1.
[f]Dipeptidyl peptidase-4.
[g]Rosiglitazone was discontinued in Europe, September 2010.

agents, the use of combinations of differently acting agents, and the introduction of insulin.

This chapter reviews new developments with existing agents, recently introduced agents and potential future agents to expand the repertoire of diabetes therapies.

8.3 New formulations

Metformin, which is the most widely prescribed oral antidiabetic agent, is prone to gastro-intestinal (GI) side effects that limit its suitability for some patients or restrict the extent of titration. A slow-release metformin formulation (Glucophage® SR in the UK, Glucophage® XR elsewhere) is now available with an extended duration of absorption. This reduces GI side effects and may enable once daily dosing with similar efficacy to twice or thrice daily standard (now termed 'immediate-release') tablets (Davidson & Howlett, 2004). The outer capsule of the slow-release formulation is not always fully degraded, which can leave an empty white 'ghost' in the faeces. To circumvent difficulties swallowing large metformin tablets there is now a liquid formulation (500 mg/5 ml), as well as sachets of a metformin powder (500 and 1000 mg) that contain aspartame as sweetener and dissolve quickly in water.

An extended-release formulation of gliclazide (Diamicron® MR) enables once-daily administration and provides increased bioavailability (Schernthaner, 2003). The 30 mg MR formulation gives similar efficacy to 80 mg of the standard formulation, and the MR formulation is said to be associated with reduced risk of hypoglycaemia and weight gain although further information is required to confirm this.

8.3.1 Single tablet combinations

Combinations of two differently acting antidiabetic agents are commonly required to achieve and sustain glycaemic targets in type 2 diabetes. Lower doses of two differently acting agents can often achieve similar or greater efficacy than a high dose of one agent, and with fewer side effects (Bailey & Day, 2009). Since diabetes patients may require a large number of medications, single-tablet 'fixed-dose' combinations can help to limit and simplify the treatment regimen, and assist compliance (Emslie-Smith et al., 2003).

Several single-tablet combinations of antidiabetic agents have been developed (Table 8.2): metformin+pioglitazone (Competact®), metformin+vildagliptin (Eucreas®) and metformin+sitagliptin (Janumet®) are approved for use in the UK (Avandamet® [metformin+ rosiglitazone] was discontinued in Europe, September 2010). Single-tablet combinations have been formulated to give bioequivalence to the two drugs administered as separate tablets. Thus they show similar efficacy and tolerability to the two active components given as separate

Table 8.2 Fixed-dose single tablet antidiabetic combinations[a,b]

Tablet®	Components	Strengths (mg)
Glucovance[f]	metformin + glibenclamide[d]	250:1.25; 500:2.5; 500-5
Metaglip[f]	metformin + glipizide	250:2.5; 500-2.5; 500-5
Avandamet[e]	metformin + rosiglitazone	500:4; 500:2; 1000:2; 1000:4
Competact[c]		
ActoplusMet[f]	metformin + pioglitazone	500:15; 850:15
Eucreas	metformin + vildagliptin	850:50; 1000:50
Janumet	metformin + sitagliptin	1000:50
PrandiMet[f]	metformin + repaglinide	500:1, 500:2
Avaglim[c, e]		
Avandaryl[e]	rosiglitazone + glimepiride	4:1; 4:2; 4:4; 8:2; 8:4
Tandemact[c, f]		
Duetact[f]	pioglitazone + glimepiride	30:2; 30:4; 45:4

[a] based on Bailey & Day (2009).
[b] availability of tablets and component strengths differ between countries.
[c] names vary between Europe and USA.
[d] glibenclamide = glyburide.
[e] Avandamet® and Avaglim®/Avandaryl® discontinued in Europe, September 2010.
[f] not available in the UK.

tablets, and require prescribers to observe the contraindications and precautions associated with each component (Bailey & Day, 2009).

8.4 Incretins (see also Figure 8.1)

Incretins are gut hormones produced during feeding to augment nutrient-induced insulin secretion. The two main incretin hormones are glucagon-like peptide-1 (GLP-1) secreted by L-cells in the ileum, and glucose-dependent insulinotropic polypeptide (GIP) secreted by K-cells in the upper small intestine. GLP-1 also potentiates the meal-related suppression of glucagon secretion, delays gastric emptying and induces satiety, and is generally associated with long-term weight loss (Holst, 2006; Drucker 2007). Both GLP-1 and GIP have been reported to increase beta-cell mass in animal studies, but this has not been confirmed in human type 2 diabetes.

8.4.1 Incretin mimetics

In type 2 diabetes the incretin effect may be diminished, due largely to impaired secretion of GLP-1. Since GLP-1 appears to retain most

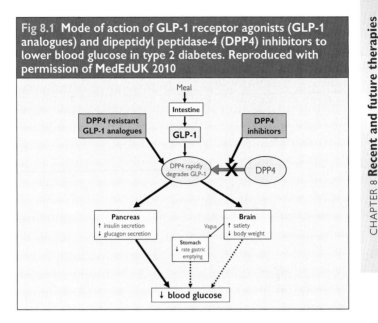

Fig 8.1 Mode of action of GLP-1 receptor agonists (GLP-1 analogues) and dipeptidyl peptidase-4 (DPP4) inhibitors to lower blood glucose in type 2 diabetes. Reproduced with permission of MedEdUK 2010

of its biological effectiveness in type 2 diabetes, administration of extra GLP-1 is a potential therapeutic approach. However GLP-1 is rapidly broken down by the enzyme dipepidyl peptidase-IV (DPP-4). Thus, to mimic the incretin effect requires DPP-4 resistant analogues of GLP-1 to act as agonists of the GLP-1 receptor. Two such agents are presently available, exenatide (Byetta®) and liraglutide (Victoza®). They are typically used as add-on therapy in obese type 2 patients who are inadequately controlled with metformin, and/or a sulfonylurea or thiazolidinedione (Flatt et al., 2009; Verspohl, 2009).

Exenatide was originally identified in saliva of the Gila monster lizard (*Heloderma suspectum*). It has 53% homology with human GLP-1 and is a full agonist of the GLP-1 receptor. An amino acid substitution (Ala8 to Gly) at the N-terminus confers resistance to degradation by DPP-4, giving a circulating half–life of about 2.4 hours (compared with ~2 min for native GLP-1) and an action duration of 4–6 hours. This allows twice daily subcutaneous injections to be given about an hour before each of the morning and evening meals. Exenatide is supplied at two doses (5 μg or 10 μg) within pre-loaded pen injectors. Treatment is usually started with the 5 μg dose *bid* for one month to reduce the risk of initial (though mostly transient) nausea, before moving to the 10 μg *bid* dose if required.

During randomized double-blind placebo controlled trials (AMIGO trials) in type 2 patients inadequately controlled with metformin and/or a sulfonylurea or thiazolidinedione, addition of exenatide reduced HbA$_{1c}$ by about 0.8–1.0% (9–11 mmol/mol) at the 10 μg dose over 6 months (DeFronzo et al., 2005; Kendall et al.,

2005; Ratner et al., 2006; Zinman et al., 2007). These effects have been sustained in open-label extension studies up to 2 years (Buse et al., 2007). The 2 hour postprandial glucose concentration was generally reduced by about 4 mmol/L, and there was little or no increase in hypoglycaemia except when add-on to a sulfonylurea. Body weight was reduced by 1.5–2.8 kg after 6 month trials with exenatide, and further weight reductions up to 5 kg occurred during open label extension studies. When compared with insulin administration in type 2 patients during trials of 6–12 months, exenatide produced similar reductions in HbA_{1c} (of about 1%; 11 mmol/mol) to biphasic insulin regimens and to basal long-acting insulin (Heine et al., 2005; Nauck et al., 2007a). Exenatide also caused weight loss whereas insulin typically caused weight gain.

Liraglutide is an analogue of GLP-1 (7–37) with an amino acid substitution (Lys34 to Arg) and a link between Lys26 to a Glu residue for attachment to a palmitoyl (C16) fatty acid chain. The latter enables the molecule to aggregate into heptamers and to attach to albumin, protecting against degradation by DPP-4 and giving a half-life of 11–15 hours. This allows once daily subcutaneous injection using a pre-loaded pen injector usually starting at 0.6 mg/day and increasing at intervals of 1–2 weeks to 1.2 and 1.8 mg/day as required.

Randomized double-blind trials with inadequately controlled type 2 diabetes patients (LEAD programme) studied liraglutide as monotherapy and as add-on to metformin and/or a sulfonylurea or thiazolidinedione. Liraglutide reduced HbA_{1c} by about 0.6–1.2% (7–13 mmol/mol) at doses of 0.6–1.8 mg/day over 6–12 months (Garber et al., 2009; Marre et al., 2009; Nauck et al., 2009; Zinman et al., 2009). Fasting plasma glucose was typically reduced by 1–2 mmol/L and postprandial glucose concentrations (measured in some studies) were reduced by about 2–3 mmol/L. There was little or no increase in hypoglycaemia, and body weight was reduced by 1–3 kg. During a 6 months trial in type 2 patients, 1.8 mg/day liraglutide produced a slightly greater reduction in HbA_{1c} (−1.33%; −14 mmol/mol) than an average 24 IU/day dose of insulin glargine (−1.09%; −12 mmol/mol) together with a reduction in body weight (Russell-Jones et al., 2009). In a 6 months head to head comparison, 1.8 mg/day liraglutide was associated with slightly greater reductions of HbA_{1c} (−1.12%; −12 mmol/mol) and mean weight reduction (−3.2 kg) than 10 ug *bid* exenatide (−0.79%; −9 mmol/mol; and −2.8 kg) (Buse et al., 2010).

GLP-1 receptor agonists delay gastric empting, thus it is recommended to avoid patients with gastroparesis and reflux, and to titrate the dose to minimize initial nausea. Consider reducing the dosage of a sulfonylurea when initiating a GLP-1 agonist, although there is low risk of serious hypoglycaemia because the insulin releasing and glucagon suppressing effects of the GLP-1 agonists do not occur at low blood glucose concentrations. GLP-1 agonists are not suitable for patients with significant renal disease and about one third of patients receiving exenatide develop antibodies, but glucose-lowering efficacy is seldom compromised. There have been reports that GLP-1 agonists are associated with acute pancreatitis, but evidence to-date suggests that the incidence is no greater than the diabetic population as a whole. GLP-1 receptors are expressed by thyroid C-cells which may account for reports of raised calcitonin levels, mostly in patients with pre-existing thyroid disease. It is interesting that many of the trials with GLP-1 agonists have noted small reductions in systolic and diastolic blood pressure, and there are preliminary reports of other potentially beneficial effects on cardiovascular function.

8.4.2 DPP-4 inhibitors

Another antihyperglycaemic strategy is to inhibit the activity of DPP-4. This will delay degradation and extend the half-lives of endogenous incretin hormones, thereby increasing the prandial insulin response (Deacon, 2004; Flatt et al., 2009; Verspohl, 2009). DPP-4 inhibitors (termed 'gliptins') are orally active, and four such agents are available in the UK: sitagliptin (Januvia®), vildagliptin (Galvus®), saxagliptin (Onglyza®) and linagliptin (Trajenta). Each is a selective inhibitor of DPP-4, and therapeutic administration has been selected to produce almost complete inhibition of circulating DPP-4 activity for >18 hours/day, increasing circulating GLP-1 concentrations by 2–3 fold. Although there are pharmacokinetic differences between the different gliptins that may affect their suitability for different sub-groups of type 2 diabetes patients (Table 8.3), the therapeutic effects of these agents appear to be very similar (Green et al., 2010).

During randomized double-blind placebo controlled trials in type 2 diabetes patients inadequately controlled with metformin, pioglitazone and/or glimepiride (mean HbA_{1c} 8.0–8.3%; 64–67 mmol/mol), addition of sitagliptin (100 mg once daily) for 6 months reduced mean HbA_{1c} by about 0.7–0.9% (7–10 mmol/mol). The addition of sitagliptin reduced the 2 hour postprandial glucose concentration by about 3 mmol/L but did not alter body weight or the occurrence of hypoglycaemia. When metformin treated patients received add-on sitagliptin compared with add-on glipizide for 1 year, each of these additional therapies reduced HbA_{1c} by about 0.7% (7 mmol/mol) but the occurrence of hypoglycaemia was much less with sitagliptin. Also, the gliptin reduced body weight (by about 1.5 kg) whereas glipizide was associated with a small weight gain (1.1 kg) (Nauck et al., 2007b).

Saxagliptin is given once daily at 5 mg, while vildagliptin is usually given as 50 mg twice daily. The similar outcomes of the three gliptins are consistent with the same mode of action (Green et al., 2010). The 2–3 fold increase in endogenous GLP-1 produced by DPP-4 inhibition is considerably less than the concentrations of injected GLP-1 analogues, which may account for a slightly lesser glucose-lowering

Table 8.3 Pharmacokinetic features of different DPP-4 inhibitors (gliptins)

	Sitagliptin	Vildagliptin	Saxagliptin	Linagliptin
Dose	100 mg od	50 mg bd	5 mg od	5 mg od
Bioavailability	~87%	~85%	50–75%	>30%
Tmax	1–4h	~1–7h	2–4h	~1.5h
Protein binding	~32%	~9%	negligible	70–80%
Metabolism	~20%, mainly liver, to very weakly active metabolites	~70% metabolized, mainly kidney to mostly inactive metabolites	~75% metabo-lized, mainly liver to active metabolites	<10% metabo-lised
Half-life	~12h	2–3h	2.5–3h	10–40h
Elimination	~80% in urine as unchanged drug	~80% in urine as metabolites	~75% in urine as metabolites	>85% in bile

effect (Pratley *et al.*, 2010). The weight neutrality observed with most studies of gliptins suggests that the increase in GLP-1 is probably not sufficient to generate the same satiety effect, but this also prevents the nausea that often accompanies injection of a GLP-1 receptor agonist.

DPP-4 degrades a variety of biologically active peptides such as bradykinin, enkephalins, gastrin releasing peptide, growth hormone-releasing hormone, insulin-like growth factor-1, neuropeptide Y, peptide YY(1–36), prolactin, substance P, several monocyte chemotactic proteins and the alpha chains of thyrotropin, luteinizing hormone and chorionic gonadotropin. However no clinically noteworthy effects of DPP-4 inhibition have been observed on vasoactivity, hunger-satiety sensations, growth, monocyte behaviour or gastrointestinal motility. DPP-4 is also the CD-26 T-cell activating antigen, but inhibition of DPP-4 peptidase activity has not been reported to affect immune function.

8.5 Pramlintide

Pramlintide (Symlin®) is a soluble analogue of amylin (islet amyloid polypeptide, IAPP). It is injected subcutaneously before meals as an adjunct to insulin therapy in type 1 or type 2 diabetes, improving glycaemic control without increasing the insulin dose. Pramlintide acts centrally, particularly via amylin receptors located in the area postrema. This activates a neurally mediated reduction in glucagon secretion, slows gastric emptying and exerts a satiety effect. The associated glucose-lowering effect frequently enables a reduction of insulin dose and a decrease in body weight (Day, 2005). The latter effect is often regarded by patients as worth the inconvenience of extra injections (pramlintide and insulin cannot be mixed in the same injection). Pramlintide is not available in Europe, but patients may read about it on the internet and ask questions.

8.6 **Other recently approved agents**

Bromocriptine and colesevelam have recently been approved by the US Food and Drug Administration to treat hyperglycaemia in type 2 diabetes.

The dopamine D_2 agonist bromocriptine, an established treatment for prolactinomas and advanced Parkinson's disease, is used at much lower doses (0.8–4.8 mg/day) for the treatment of type 2 diabetes. A quick-release formulation administered early after waking appears to act centrally to raise dopaminergic activity in several brain centres including the hypothalamus. Evidence to-date suggests that the morning burst of dopaminergic activity acts in synchrony with serotoninergic activity to regularize circadian rhythmicity of hypothalamic nuclei involved in the peripheral control of glucose homeostasis (Gaziano et al., 2010; Scranton & Cincotta, 2010). In 4–12 month trials with type 2 diabetes patients, the quick-release bromocriptine (Cycloset), given as monotherapy or in combination with other diabetes medications, reduced HbA_{1c} by 0.6–1.2% (6–13 mmol/mol). The effect occurred without raising insulin levels or body weight, and there was low risk of hypoglycaemia. Although some patients reported nausea the drug was well tolerated at the low doses and blood pressure was slightly reduced in some patients. The doses of bromocriptine were considered low enough to avoid retroperitoneal fibrosis or disturbances of heart valves seen at much higher doses.

In addition to its use as a bile acid sequestrant in the treatment of hypercholesterolaemia, colesevelam is indicated in the USA to assist glucose-lowering in diabetes patients. When studied for 6 months in type 2 patients as monotherapy or add-on to metformin +/- other oral antidiabetes agents, colesevelam (six tablets daily of 625mg) reduced HbA_{1c} by about 0.5% (5–6 mmol/mol). There was little change in C-peptide or body weight, low risk of hypoglycaemia and lipid parameters were improved. Since the sequestrant is not absorbed there has been speculation that the glucose-lowering effect might be associated with an effect on bile acid recirculation, hepatic cholesterol handling or GLP-1 secretion (Bays et al., 2008).

8.7 **Future antidiabetic therapies**

A once-weekly depot injection of exenatide is now available in many countries including the USA and UK and several other GLP-1 agonists are presently in phase 3 clinical trial (Kim *et al.*, 2007; Flatt *et al.*, 2009). One such GLP-1 agonist in phase 3 development is lixisenatide. This is a once daily GLP-1 agonist with the advantages of its class with weight loss and low risk of hypoglycaemia. It has a particularly marked effect on postprandial plasma glucose providing a particular rationale for combination with long-acting basal insulin analogues to further improve glycaemic control without increased risk of hypoglycaemia or weight gain. Combination (hybrid) peptides are at an early stage of development: for example, part of the GLP-1 sequence that retains GLP-1 agonist activity has been linked with part of the glucagon sequence that is a competitive antagonist at the glucagon receptor. These hybrid peptides appear able to potentiate glucose-induced insulin secretion and reduce glucagon action.

Inhibitors of the renal sodium-glucose cotransporter-2 (SGLT2) increase the elimination of excess glucose in the urine, offering a novel insulin independent mechanism to lower blood glucose (Bailey & Day, 2010) (Figure 8.2). The most advanced in development is dapagliflozin. A 10 mg once-daily dose of this agent reduced HbA$_{1c}$ by 0.54% (6 mmol/mol) when given to type 2 patients for 6 months as add-on therapy to metformin (Bailey *et al.*, 2010). There was no

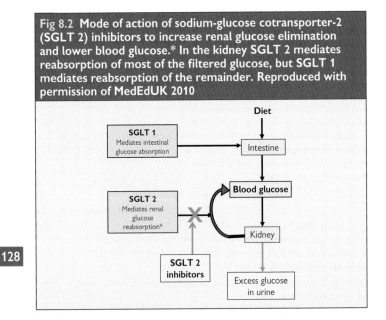

Fig 8.2 **Mode of action of sodium-glucose cotransporter-2 (SGLT 2) inhibitors to increase renal glucose elimination and lower blood glucose.* In the kidney SGLT 2 mediates reabsorption of most of the filtered glucose, but SGLT 1 mediates reabsorption of the remainder. Reproduced with permission of MedEdUK 2010**

increased risk of hypoglycaemia, body weight was reduced by about 2 kg and systolic blood pressure was reduced by 5 mmHg.

Glucokinase activators can enhance glucose-induced insulin secretion and increase hepatic glucose uptake and metabolism. These agents will require careful dose titration to avoid episodes of hypoglycaemia, and are currently being evaluated to treat type 2 diabetes. Tissue-specific reduction of active glucocorticoids is being assessed as a means of reducing blood glucose and body weight by inhibiting the cortisone-activating enzyme 11-beta hydroxysteroid dehydrogenase-1. Selective modulators of peroxisome proliferator-activated receptors are also receiving clinical investigation. These and other potential new types of glucose-lowering agents are reviewed in detail elsewhere (Barnett & Bailey 2007; Bailey 2009).

8.8 Conclusion

Several additions to the antidiabeic armamentarium have recently emerged. These include new formulations of established drugs to improve tolerability, single tablet 'fixed-dose' combinations to reduce the pill burden, a longer-acting GLP-1 agonist, DPP-4 inhibitors with different pharmacokinetic features, and agents previously used for other purposes (such as quick-release bromocriptine). The choice of therapies for type 2 diabetes is therefore expanding to meet the need for improved glycaemic control.

References

Bailey CJ (2009) New therapies for diabesity *Curr. Diabetes Reps* **9**: 360–7.

Bailey CJ, Day C (2009) Fixed-dose single tablet antidiabetic combinations. *Diabetes Obes Metab* **11**: 527–33.

Bailey CJ, Day C (2010) SGLT2 inhibitors: glucuretic treatment for type 2 diabetes. *Br J Diabetes Vasc Dis* **10**: 193–9.

Bailey CJ, Gross JL, Pieters A, et al. (2010) Effect of dapagliflozin in patients with type 2 diabetes who have inadequate glycaemic control with metformin: a randomized, double-blind, placebo-controlled trial. *Lancet* **375**: 2223–33.

Barnett AH (2011) Lixisenatide: evidence for its potential use in the treatment of type 2 diabetes. *Core Evidence* **6**: 1–13.

Barnett AH, Bailey CJ (eds) (2007) *Best Practice and Research: Clinical Endocrinology & Metabolism* **21**: 497–710. (Elsevier)

Bays HE, Goldberg RB, Ruitt KE, Jones MR (2008) Colesevelam hydrochloride therapy in patients with type 2 diabetes mellitus treated with metformin. *Arch Intern Med* **168**: 1975–83.

Buse JB, Klonoff DC, Nielsen LL, et al. (2007) Metabolic effects of two years of exenatide treatment on diabetes, obesity, and hepatic biomarkers in patients with type 2 diabetes: an interim analysis of data from the open label, uncontrolled extension of three double-blind, placebo-controlled trials. *Clin Ther* **29**; 139–53.

Buse JB, Rosenstock J, Sesti G, *et al.* (2010) Liraglutide once a day versus exenatide twice a day for type 2 diabetes: a 28 week randomised, parallel-group. multinational, open-label trial (Lead-8). *Lancet* **374**: 39–47.

Davidson J, Howlett HCS (2004) New prolonged release metformin improves gastrointestinal tolerability. *Br J Diabetes Vasc Dis* **4**: 273–7.

Day C (2005) Amylin analogue as an antidiabetic. *Br J Diabetes Vasc Dis* **5**: 151–4.

Deacon CF (2004) Therapeutic strategies based on glucagon-like peptide-1. *Diabetes* **53**: 2181–9.

DeFronzo RA, Ratner RE, Han J, Kim DD, Fineman MS, Baron AD (2005) Effects of exenatide (exendin-4) on glycemic control and weight over 30 weeks in metformin treated patients with type 2 diabetes. *Diabetes Care* **28**: 1092–1100.

Drucker DJ (2007) The role of gut hormones in glucose homeostasis. *J Clin Invest* **117**: 24–32.

Emslie-Smith A, Dowall J, Morris AD (2003) The problem of polypharmacy in type 2 diabetes. *Br J Diabetes Vasc Dis* **3**: 54–6.

Flatt PR, Bailey CJ, Green BD (2009) Recent advances in antidiabetic drug therapies targeting the enteroinsular axis. *Curr Drug Metabolism* **10**: 125–37.

Garber A, Henry R, Ratner, *et al.* (2009) Liraglutide versus glimepiride mono-therapy for type 2 diabetes (LEAD-3 mono): A randomised, 52-week, phase III, double-blind, parallel-treatment trial. *Lancet* **373**: 473–81.

Gaziano JM, Cincotta AH, O'Connor CM, *et al.* (2010) Randomised clinical trial of quick-release bromocriptine among patients with type 2 diabetes on overall safety and cardiovascular outcomes. *Diabetes Care* **33**: 1503–8.

Green BD, Bailey CJ, Flatt PR (2010) Gliptin therapies for inhibiting dipeptidyl peptidase-4 in type 2 diabetes. *European Endocrinol.* **5**: 2–8.

Heine RJ, Van Gaal LF, Johns D, *et al.* (2005) Exenatide versus insulin glargine in patients with suboptimally controlled type 2 diabetes: a randomized trial. *Ann Intern Med* **143**: 59–69.

Holst JJ (2006) Glucagon-like peptide-1: from extract to agent. *Diabetologia* **49**: 253–60.

Kendall DM, Riddle MC, Rosenstock J, *et al.* (2005) Effects of exenatide (Exendin-4) on glycemic control over 30 weeks in patients with type 2 diabetes treated with metformin and a sulfonylurea. *Diabetes Care* **28**: 1083–91.

Kim D, Macconell L, Zhuang D, *et al.* (2007) Effects of once weekly dosing of a long-acting release formulation of exenatide on glucose control and body weight in subjects with type 2 diabetes. *Diabetes Care* **30**: 1487–93.

Krentz AJ, Bailey CJ (2005) Oral antidiabetic agents. Current role in type 2 diabetes mellitus. *Drugs* **65**: 385–411.

Marre M, Shaw J, Brandle M, *et al.* (2009) Lriglutide, a once-daily human GLP-1 analogue, added to a sulphonylurea over 26 weeks produces greater improvements in glycaemic control and weight control compared with adding rosiglitazone or placebo in subjects with type 2 diabetes (LEAD-1 SU). *Diabetic Med* **26**: 268–78.

Nathan DM, Buse JB, Davidson MB, et al. (2009) Medical management of hyperglycaemia in type 2 diabetes: a consensus algorithm for the initiation and adjustment of therapy. A consensus statement of the American Diabetes Association and the European Association for the Study of Diabetes Diabetologia. *Diabetes Care* **52**: 17–30.

Nauck MA, Frid A, Hermansen K, et al. (2009) Efficacy and safety coparison of liraglutide, glimepiride and placebo, all in combination with metformin in type 2 diabetes: the LEAD 2 study. *Diabetes Care* **32**: 84–90.

Nauck MA, Duran S, Kim D, et al. (2007a) A comparison of twice-daily exenatide and biphasic insulin aspart in patients with type 2 diabetes who were suboptimally controlled with sulfonylurea and metformin: a non-inferiority study. *Diabetologia* **50**: 259–67.

Nauck MA, Meininger G Sheng D, et al. (2007b) Efficacy and safety of the dipeptidyl peptidase-4 inhibitor sitagliptin compared with the sulphonylurea glipizide inpatients with type 2 diabetes inadequately controlled on metformin alone. *Diabetes Obesity Metab.* **9**: 194–205.

Pratley RE, Nauck M, Bailey T, et al. (2010) Liraglutide versus sitagliptin for patients with type 2 diabetes who did not have adequate glycaemic control with metformin: a 26-week, randomised, parallel-group, open-label trial. *Lancet* **375**: 1447–56.

Ratner RE, Maggs D, Nielsen, et al. (2006) Long-term effects of exenatide therapy over 82 weeks on glycaemic control and weight in over-weight metformin-treated patients with type 2 diabetes mellitus. *Diabetes Obes Metab* **8**: 419–28.

Russell-Jones D, Vaag A, Schmidtz O, et al. (2009) Lirgalutide vs insulin glargine and placebo in combination with metformin and sulphonylurea therapy in type 2 diabetes mellitus (LEAD-5 met+SU): a randomised controlled trial. *Diabetologia* **52**: 2046–55.

Schernthaner G (2003) Gliclazide modified release: a critical review of pharmacodynamic, metabolic and vasoprotective effects. *Metabolism* **52**: 29–34.

Scranton R, Cincotta A (2010) Bromocriptine—unique formulation of a dopamine agonist for the treatment of type 2 diabetes. *Expert Opinion Pharmacother* **11**: 269–79.

Verspohl EJ (2009) Novel therapeutics for type 2 diabetes: incretin hormone mimetics (glucagon-like peptide-2 receptor agonists) and dipeptidyl peptidase-4 inhibitors. *Pharmacol Therapeutics* **124**: 113–38.

Zinman B, Gerich J, Buse J, et al. (2009) Efficacy and safety of the GLP-1 analog liraglutide in combination with metformin and TZD in patients with type 2 diabetes mellitus (LEAD-4 Met+TZD). *Diabetes Care* **32**: 1224–30.

Zinman B, Hoogwerf BJ, Garcia SD, et al. (2007) The effect of adding exenatide to a thiazolidinedione in suboptimally controlled type 2 diabetes. *Ann Intern Med* **146**: 477–85.

Chapter 9

Management of type 2 diabetes and insulin

Rajesh Peter, Richard A Chudleigh, David R Owens and Anthony Barnett

> **Key points**
> - Since type 2 diabetes is a progressive disease many patients will eventually require insulin therapy
> - Initiation of insulin is often inappropriately delayed resulting in adverse health consequences
> - Several different types of insulin are available and the regime used should be tailored to the needs of the individual patient, but informed by recent clinical trial data
> - Early and efffective use of insulin will commonly improve symptoms and help to achieve better glycaemic control thereby reducing the risk of longterm vascular complications.

133

9.1 Introduction

The prevalence of type 2 diabetes (T2DM) and its vascular complications has reached epidemic proportions and promises to continue unabated, fuelled by the parallel increase in obesity, a more sedentary lifestyle and increasing longevity especially in developed countries. In a large study one in five (21%) deaths from ischaemic heart disease and 1 in 8 (13%) from stroke were attributable to higher than optimum blood glucose levels (Danaei *et al.*, 2006). It is also now recognized that achieving improved glycaemic control can consequently reduce morbidity and mortality (EDPG, 1999; ADA, 2005). There are various categories of medications that can lower glycaemia, with insulin being the oldest and still the most effective. Insulin therapy in T2DM is most commonly reserved for patients in whom a trial of lifestyle intervention and/or oral hypoglycaemic agents therapy has failed to achieve glycaemic targets (fasting blood glucose, HbA_{1c} and more latterly postprandial glucose). Historically, instituting insulin therapy is unnecessarily delayed due to a variety of reasons including patient reluctance because of fear of hypoglycaemia or ignorance about benefits of good glycaemic control, perceived complexity and time constraints of initiating insulin by healthcare professionals. Based on the natural history of T2DM, given time most patients will eventually require therapy with insulin. The time period before insulin is required depends on various factors including the rate of islet β cell failure, extent of hyperglycaemia (concept of glucotoxicity), degree of obesity (insulin resistance), concomitant medications and a variety of illnesses that may exacerbate the insulin need. The many types of insulins and regimens available today means that the current situation is relatively complex for many healthcare professionals, in contrast to the management of hypercholesterolemia and possibly hypertension.

Though insulin was initially developed to treat type 1 diabetes, in whom it is life saving, its potential value in treating other types of diabetes was recognized early on by Himmsworth and Kerr (Himmsworth & Kerr, 1939). The beneficial use of insulin in such patients, later referred to as T2DM, emerged many years later from a number of long term large scale clinical trials. In the UKPDS (UKPDS, 1998), 3867 newly diagnosed subjects with T2DM were randomized to a conventionally treated arm, i.e. dietary treatment and aiming for a FPG <15 mmol/l (n=1138) and an intensively treated arm comprising of either a sulfonylurea (n=1573) or insulin (n=1156) aiming for a FPG <6 mmol/l. After 10 years the HbA_{1c} achieved in the intensive treated group was 7.0% (6.2–8.2) compared with 7.9% (6.9–8.8) in the conventional group resulting in a 25% risk reduction (95% CI 7–40; $p=0.0099$) in microvascular endpoints. There was no difference between insulin and sulfonylureas. In the prospective observational arm of the study each 1% reduction in HbA_{1c} was also associated with a 14% reduction in myocardial infarction (95% CI 8–21; $p<0.0001$) (Stratton et al., 2000). In the Kumamoto study (Ohkubo et al., 1995), n=110 patients with T2DM were randomly assigned to multiple insulin injection treatment (MIT)—i.e. short-acting insulin at each meal and intermediate-acting insulin at bedtime or to conventional insulin treatment (CIT)—i.e. 1 or 2 daily injections of intermediate-acting insulin. The mean HbA_{1c} over 6 years was significantly ($p<0.001$) lower in the MIT group than in the CIT group (7.1±1.1 vs. 9.4±1.5%). After 6 years the development of retinopathy was 7.7% in the MIT group and 32.0% for the CIT group in the primary prevention cohort ($p=0.039$) and progression of diabetic retinopathy was 19.2% in the MIT group and 44.0% in the CIT group ($p=0.049$). The development of nephropathy was 7.7% in the MIT group and 28.0% for the CIT group in the primary prevention cohort ($p=0.032$) and progression of nephropathy was 11.5% and 32.0% for the MIT and CIT groups respectively, in the secondary intervention cohort ($p=0.044$). There was also a ~50% reduction in macrovascular complications but the results did not reach statistical significance as the sample size was small.

In the landmark Steno-2 trial (Gaede et al., 2003), 160 people with T2DM and microalbuminuria were randomized to conventional treatment or intensive treatment with lifestyle modification and pharmacological interventions. Hyperglycaemia, hypertension, dys-lipidaemia, microalbuminuria, and prevention of CVD with aspirin were targeted in the intensive treatment arm. Hyperglycaemia in the intensive treatment arm was addressed by a stepwise introduction of pharmacologic therapy. Patients unable to maintain HbA_{1c} <6.5% with diet and exercise were started on oral hypoglycaemic agents. Those patients with HbA_{1c} >7%, despite maximal doses of oral agents were given neutral protamine Hagedorn (NPH) insulin (isophane insulin) at bedtime, and if daily dose exceeded 80 units at bedtime or there was no change in HbA_{1c}, regular insulin was given along with NPH insulin 2 to 4 times a day. Over the 7.8 years of follow up, it was found that patients receiving intensive therapy had a significantly lower risk of CVD (hazard ratio 0.47; 95% CI 0.24 to 0.73; $p=0.008$), nephropathy (hazard ratio 0.39; 95% CI 0.17 to 0.87; $p=0.003$) and retinopathy (hazard ratio 0.42; 95% CI 0.21 to 0.86; $p=0.02$) compared to the conventionally treated group.

9.2 **Insulin preparations**

Insulin therapy has progressed over the years. For the first 50 years, bovine and porcine insulin was in widespread clinical use. In the early 1980s human insulin became a commercial reality. Insulin analogues which are produced by recombinant DNA technology have now gained wider acceptance due to their physical and chemical proper-ties. Insulin preparations available to control blood glucose include:

- fast-acting insulin analogues (aspart, lispro, glulisine)
- short-acting preparations (regular human insulin)
- intermediate-acting insulins (NPH, Lente insulins, insulin detemir)
- long-acting insulins (Ultralente, insulin glargine)
- insulin mixtures (Novomix® 30/70, Humalog® Mix 25/75, Human Mixtard®, 50/50).

9.3 **Achieving glycaemic control in T2DM**

The primary goal in glycaemia management in type 2 diabetes is achieving and maintaining glucose levels as close to the nondiabetic range as possible. A joint consensus statement from the ADA/EASD was recently published as a guide for the initiation and adjustment of therapy in patients with type 2 diabetes (Nathan *et al.*, 2006). An important message in this consensus statement was the need for rapid addition of medications and transition to new regimens when glycaemic goals were not achieved or sustained and also the early introduction of insulin therapy in patients who do not meet target goals. Where lifestyle intervention and metformin (and a second oral hypoglycaemic agent) do not achieve glycaemic targets, insulin initiation would be one of the next options along with sulfonylureas and the thiazolidenediones group of drugs. In general, earlier and more aggressive management of patients to glycaemic targets is advocated without placing the patient at risk of hypoglycaemia or acceleration of microvascular complications eg. diabetic retinopathy in subjects with long-term poor glycaemic control and evidence of diabetic retinopathy in whom a more gradual improvement in glycaemic control is essential.

9.4 **Introduction of insulin in T2DM**

There are several acceptable methods to initiate insulin therapy but a consensus opinion on how to initiate insulin treatment in subjects with T2DM is lacking. A regimen that is easy to apply and is as efficacious as another with minimal resulting hypoglycaemic attacks would be the ideal regimen. Commonly used insulin initiation strategies include:

• basal insulin in addition to oral agents
• premixed biphasic analogues in addition to oral agents
• basal plus prandial insulin up to full basal bolus therapy.

A popular regimen is to initiate once a day long or intermediate acting insulin at night. The Treat-To-Target Study (Riddle *et al.*, 2003) demonstrated the ease of administration and effectiveness of combination therapy with oral agents during the day and 1 injection of insulin glargine or isophane (NPH) insulin given at night in ~750 patients (age ~55 years, BMI ~32, duration of diabetes ~8.5 years). After 24 weeks of combination therapy, the average HbA_{1c} for the two groups decreased from 8.6% to <7.0% using an aggressive titration schedule. The study used a starting dose of 10 IU of insulin glargine with forced weekly titration algorithm to achieve FPG <5.6 mmol/l. Both treatment arms were equally effective, however, nearly 25% more patients attained this without documented nocturnal hypoglycaemia in the insulin glargine group. The incidence of severe hypoglycaemia was uncommon in both groups occurring in ~2% of patients. Similar advantages with insulin glargine were also observed in other studies (Yki-Jarvinen *et al.*, 2000; Rosenstock *et al.*, 2001) while being as efficacious as isophane (NPH) insulin. In the LANMET study (Yki-Jarvinen *et al.*, 2006) n=110 insulin naive subjects with T2DM with HbA$_{1c}$ >8.0% on oral hypoglycaemic agents were randomized to receive bedtime insulin glargine with metformin (G+MET) [mean HbA$_{1c}$ 9.5 ± 0.1] or bedtime NPH (isophane insulin) with metformin (NPH+MET) [mean HbA$_{1c}$ 9.6 ± 0.1]. After 36 weeks HbA$_{1c}$ was 7.14 ± 0.12 and 7.16 ± 0.14% (*p*=NS) in the G+MET and NPH+MET groups, respectively. Symptomatic hypoglycaemia during the first 12 weeks was significantly lower in the G+MET group at 4.1 ± 0.8 episodes/patient-year than in the NPH+MET group at 9.0 ± 2.3 episodes/patient-year (*p*<0.05).

Traditionally FPG and HbA$_{1c}$ have been used to guide insulin titration. Also patient adjusted titration algorithms aiming for similar FPG targets can achieve comparable improvements in HbA$_{1c}$ to physician adjusted algorithms (Davies *et al.*, 2005). This regime involving one daily injection can be easily titrated and achieves target HbA$_{1c}$ in the majority of patients (up to approximately 60%). This regime has also been shown to work favourably for group insulin initiation as was shown by the INITIATE study (Yki-Jarvinen *et al.*, 2007). In this multicentre, two arm parallel design study insulin naïve subjects with T2DM with an HbA$_{1c}$ of 7.0–12.0% were randomized to initiate bedtime insulin glargine either individually or in groups of 4–8. The total time spent in initiating insulin was 4.2 ± 0.2 hours and 2.2 ± 0.2 hours respectively. After 24 weeks HbA$_{1c}$ decreased from 8.7 ± 0.2 to 6.9 ± 0.1%, and from 8.8 ± 0.2 to 6.8 ± 0.1% (*p*=NS) in the individually treated and those treated in groups respectively with similar treatment satisfaction scores.

The importance of postprandial glucose on overall glycaemia has been demonstrated in a few studies (Monnier *et al.*, 2003; Peter *et al.*, 2006) with the contribution of postprandial glucose being predominant in those subjects with HbA$_{1c}$ <~8.0%. Hence the addition of a fast acting insulin component to a basal regimen may allow more patients to achieve recommended glycaemic targets by further controlling postprandial glucose. Another approach to starting insulin is to initiate one or two injections of premixed insulin containing a fixed ratio of either regular or fast-acting insulin analogue and intermediate-acting insulin. In a study by Raskin *et al.* (Raskin *et al.*, 2005) n=233 insulin naïve patients poorly controlled on oral hypoglycaemic agents were randomized to either twice daily biphasic insulin aspart 30/70 (BIAsp 30/70) or once daily insulin glargine and doses titrated to achieve FPG and pre-supper plasma glucose values of 4.4–6.1 mmol/l (age ~52 years, BMI 31, duration of diabetes ~9 years). After 28 weeks, initiating insulin therapy with BIAsp 30/70 was more effective in lowering HbA$_{1c}$ compared to once daily glargine −2.79 ± 0.11 vs −2.36 ± 0.11% (*p*<0.01) respectively. The HbA$_{1c}$ reductions were mainly accounted for in subjects whose baseline HbA$_{1c}$ values were

>8.5%: −3.13 ± 1.63 vs −2.60 ± 1.50% ($p<0.05$). In subjects with base-line HbA_{1c} <8.5%, absolute HbA_{1c} reductions did not differ between the two treatment groups −1.40 ± 0.53 vs −1.42 ± 0.59% ($p>0.05$). Episodes of hypoglycaemia [episodes/year] 3.4 ± 6.6 vs 0.7 ± 2.0 ($p<0.05$) and weight gain 5.4 ± 4.8 vs 3.5 ± 4.5 kg ($p<0.01$) were greater in the BIAsp 30/70 treated subjects than for glargine treated subjects respectively. In another study (Janka et al., 2005), therapy with once daily glargine added to oral hypoglycaemic agents was compared with twice daily biphasic human insulin premix alone. Initiating insulin treatment by adding basal insulin glargine once daily to ongoing oral hypoglycaemic therapy was more effective (mean HbA_{1c} decrease from baseline %) −1.64, 95% CI −1.51 to −1.78 vs −1.31, 95% CI −1.17 to −1.44 ($p=0.0003$) and safer than beginning twice daily injections of biphasic insulin premix and discontinuing oral hypoglycaemic agents. Many reasons have been cited for the discrepancy in the results between this study and the study by Raskin et al. (Raskin et al., 2005) including the use of aspart an insulin analogue with a more rapid onset of action resulting in better postprandial glucose control and also that oral hypoglycaemic agents were stopped in the insulin premix arm in the study by Janka et al. (Janka et al., 2005).

Many patients are not considered for insulin therapy until HbA_{1c} levels are very much higher than the target of 7.0%. Mean HbA_{1c} levels of 10.4% were reported in one cohort (Haywood et al., 1997) commencing insulin therapy. In another study it was hypotheti-cally estimated that patients carried an excess of 10 HbA_{1c}–years of burden >7.0% from diagnosis until starting insulin (Brown et al., 2004). Moreover those patients who fail to achieve target HbA_{1c} with basal insulin are usually those with poor baseline HbA_{1c} i.e. >8.5% or those who are insulin resistant requiring insulin doses >0.5 U/kg. In these types of patients, glycaemic targets will not usually be achieved with basal insulin alone. As yet no consensus exists as to which insulin regime should be employed in this setting. One option is to convert these patients to twice daily biphasic insulin premix, and a small minority may even need it three times a day. Another option, discussed subsequently is addition of prandial insulin targeting the largest daily postprandial excursion. This strategy may ultimately lead to the classical basal bolus regime. This regime allows great-est flexibility and a stepwise addition of prandial insulin. Generally sulfonylureas would be stopped if biphasic insulin premix or prandial insulin is chosen. It has been shown that continuing administration of sulfonylureas with these regimens may expose patients to additional hypoglycaemic risk and thereby limit insulin dose adjustment, thus providing little or no additional benefit at this stage of the disease (Yki-Jarvinen et al., 1999).

The third strategy is to target postprandial glucose using prandial insulin. The Treat to Target in Type 2 Diabetes (4-T) (Holman et al.,

2007) is a 3-year multicentre, open label, randomized control clinical trial comparing the efficacy and safety of adding analogue biphasic insulin, prandial or basal insulin to (n=708) subjects with T2DM (age ~62 years, BMI ~30, duration of diabetes ~9.0 years) with suboptimal glycaemic control (HbA$_{1c}$ ~8.5%) while receiving maximally tolerated doses of metformin and sulfonylurea. At 1 year, HbA$_{1c}$ levels were similar (p=0.08) in the biphasic group (7.3%) and the prandial group (7.2%) but significantly higher (p<0.001 for both comparisons) in the basal group (7.6%). The number of hypoglycaemic events were 5.7, 12.0 and 2.3 (per patient per year) and mean weights were 4.7, 5.7, and 1.9 kg respectively. The dosing and titration algorithm for insulin is just as important as the type of insulin chosen. The study aimed to lower patient's HbA$_{1c}$ to ≤6.5%, however disappointingly, only a minority of patients achieved the target goal (17% in the biphasic group, 24% in the prandial group and 8% in the basal group). It is possible that the treatment algorithm was insufficiently proactive. This study showed that in patients suboptimally controlled (mean HbA$_{1c}$ ~8.5%) on oral hypoglycaemic agents the addition of biphasic and prandial insulins reduced HbA$_{1c}$ more than the addition of basal insulin but with greater weight gain and a higher risk of hypoglycaemia. This study inferred that T2DM patients may need more than one type of insulin to achieve their target blood glucose levels, and this has since been confirmed by the findings from this trial at 3 years—over 80% of patients initiated on basal insulin subsequently required a second-line type of insulin to maintain good glycaemic control (Holman et al., 2009).

If despite FPG <5.6 mmol/l being achieved and HbA$_{1c}$ remains above target or basal insulin dose exceeds 0.5–0.7 U/kg consider adding prandial insulin* and stopping the insulin secretagogue.

Insulin detemir—if pre-dinner BG >6.1 mmol/l add second dose of detemir in the morning. See also Box 9.1, and Tables 9.1 and 9.2.

Box 9.1 Algorithm for initiation of insulin in patients with type 2 diabetes

Initiation of basal insulin in subjects with HbA$_{1c}$ <8.5% on metformin and/or an insulin secretagogue.

1 Start insulin glargine/detemir at a dose of 10 U at bed time

2 Insulin dose to be titrated to achieve a pre-breakfast fasting blood glucose of <5.6 mmol/l, according to the algorithm taken from the treat to target trial# (Riddle et al., 2003).

#Other titration algorithms are also available (AT.LANTUS study group).

---

*Rapid acting prandial insulin can be added to basal insulin glargine/detemir, targeting the main daily postprandial glucose excursion (aiming for 2 hour post-breakfast plasma glucose <10.0 mmol/l, post-lunch <7.8 mmol/l and post-dinner <10 mmol/l) or change to a pre-mixed biphasic regime twice a day initially, with some patients requiring additional soluble insulin or a third dose of the premixed biphasic insulin at mid-day meal.

Table 9.1 Dose titration algorithm for basal insulin (insulin glargine) from Riddle MC, et al. (2003); The Treat-to-Target Trial

Mean of self monitored FBG values from preceding 2 days	Increase of insulin dose (U/day)
≥10 mmol/l	8
7.8–10 mmol/l	6
6.7–7.8 mmol/l	4
5.6–6.7 mmol/l	2

No increase in dose if a plasma reference (meter adjusted) range value <4.0 was documented during the previous week.

A small decrease in dose (2–4 U) allowed if severe hypoglycaemia or a plasma reference range value of <3.1 mmol/l were documented in the previous week.

In subjects with HbA$_{1c}$ levels of >8.5% treated with metformin and an insulin secretagogue, early use of a basal plus prandial insulin or premixed biphasic insulin should be considered (at commencement of prandial insulin, secretagogues are conventionally discontinued).

9.5 Conclusion

It is now generally accepted that achieving good glycaemic control reduces morbidity and mortality. Initiating insulin therapy is often delayed due to various reasons and the resulting glycaemic burden

Table 9.2 Dose titration algorithm for premixed insulin from the Raskin et al study (2005)

Start with 10–12 U of biphasic insulin pre-breakfast and pre-supper			
Fasting blood glucose for 3 consecutive days	Adjust pre supper insulin dose (IU/day)	Presupper glucose concentration for 3 consecutive days	Adjust pre breakfast insulin dose (IU/day)
>9.9 mmol/l	6	>9.9 mmol/l	6
7.8–9.9 mmol/l	4	7.8–9.9 mmol/l	4
6.1–7.8 mmol/l	2	6.1–7.8 mmol/l	2
4.4–6.1 mmol/l	No change	4.4–6.1 mmol/l	No change
3.3–4.4 mmol/l	−2	3.3–4.4 mmol/l	−2
<3.3 #	−4	<3.3	−4

If a single reading in this range make appropriate dose adjustment.

is considerable. Various insulins are utilized to control blood glucose with emerging data comparing the different options. If the epidemic of diabetes and its complications is to be reduced, early and effective use of insulin is paramount.

References

American Diabetes Association (2005) Standards of medical care of diabetes. *Diabetes Care* **28**: S15–S35.

Brown JB, Nichols GA, Perry A (2004) The burden of treatment failure in type 2 diabetes. *Diabetes Care* **27**: 1535–40.

Danaei G, Lawes CMM, Hoom SV, Murray CJ, Ezzati M (2006) Global and regional mortality from ischaemic heart disease and stroke attributable to higher than optimum blood glucose concentration: comparative risk assessment. *Lancet* **368**: 1651–9.

Davies M, Storms F, Shutler S, Bianchi-Biscay M, Gomis R (2005) Improvement of glycaemic control in subjects with poorly controlled type 2 diabetes. Comparison of two treatment algorithms using insulin glargine. *Diabetes Care* **28**: 1282–8.

European Diabetes Policy Group (1999) A desk-top guide to type 2 diabetes mellitus. *Diabetic Med* **16**: 716–30.

Gaede P, Vedel P, Larsen N, Jensen GV, Parving HH, Pedersen O (2003) Multifactorial intervention and cardiovascular disease in patients with type 2 diabetes. *NEJM* **348**: 383–93.

Haywood RA, Manning WG, Kaplan SH, Wagner EH, Greenfield S (1997) Starting insulin therapy in patients with type 2 diabetes: effectiveness, complications and resource utilization. *JAMA* **278**: 1663–9.

Himmsworth HP, Kerr RB (1939) Insulin sensitive and insulin insensitive types of diabetes mellitus. *Clin Sci* **4**: 119–52.

Holman RR, Thorne KI, Farmer AJ, Davies MJ, Keenan JF, Paul SP, Levy JC (2007) Addition of biphasic, prandial or basal insulin to oral therapy in type 2 diabetes. *N Engl J Med* **357**: 1716–30.

Holman RR, Farmer AJ, Davies MJ, *et al.* (2009) Three year efficacy of complex insulin regimens in type 2 diabetes. *N Eng J Med* **361**: 1736–47.

Janka HU, Plewe G, Riddle MC, Kliebe-Frisch C, Schweitzer MA, Yki-Jarvinen H (2005) Comparison of basal insulin added to oral agents versus twice daily pre-mixed insulin as initial insulin therapy for type 2 diabetes. *Diabetes Care* **28**: 254–9.

Monnier L, Lapinski H, Colette C (2003) Contributions of fasting and post-prandial plasma glucose increments to the overall diurnal hyperglycaemia of type 2 diabetic patients. *Diabetes Care* **26**: 881–5.

Nathan DM, Buse JB, Davidson MB, Heine RJ, Holman RR, Sherwin R, Zinman B (2006) Management of hyperglycaemia in type 2 diabetes: A consensus algorithm for the initiation and adjustment of therapy. *Diabetes Care* **29**: 1963–72.

Ohkubo Y, Kishikawa H, Araki E, Miyata T, Isami S, Motoyoshi S, Kojima Y, Furuyoshi N, Shichiri M (1995) Intensive insulin therapy prevents the pregression of diabetic microvascular complications in Japanese patients with non-insulin dependant diabetes mellitus: a randomised prospective 6-year study. *Diabetes Res Clin Pract* **28**: 103–17.

Peter R, Luzio SD, Dunseath G, Pauvaday V, Owens DR (2006) Relationship between HbA$_{1c}$ and indices of glucose tolerance derived from a standardized meal test in newly diagnosed treatment naïve subjects with type 2 diabetes. *Diabetic Medicine* **23**: 990–5.

Raskin P, Allen E, Hollander P, Lewin A, Gabbay RA, Hu P, Bode B, Garber A (2005) Initiating insulin therapy in type 2 diabetes. A comparison of biphasic and basal insulin analogs. *Diabetes Care* **28**: 260–5.

Riddle MC, Rosenstock J, Gerich J (2003) The treat-to-target trial. *Diabetes Care* **26**: 3080–6.

Rosenstock J, Schwartz SL, Clark CM, Park GD, Donley DW, Edwards MB (2001) Basal insulin therapy in type 2 diabetes. *Diabetes Care* **24**: 631–6.

Stratton I, Adler AI, Neil HAW, *et al.* (2000) Association of glycaemia with macrovascular and microvascular complications of type 2 diabetes (UKPDS 35): prospective observational study. *BMJ* **321**: 405–12.

UK prospective Diabetes Study (UKPDS) Group (1998) Intensive blood glucose control with sulphonylureas or insulin compared with conventional treatment and risk of complications in patients with type 2 diabetes (UKPDS 33). *Lancet* **352**: 837–53.

Yki-Jarvinen H, Ryysy L, Nikkila K, Tulokas T, Vanamo R, Heikkila M (1999) Comparison of bedtime insulin regimens in patients with type 2 diabetes mellitus: a randomised, controlled trial. *Ann Intern Med* **130**: 389–96.

Yki-Jarvinen H, Dressler A, Ziemen M (2000) Less nocturnal hypoglycaemia and better post-dinner glucose control with bedtime insulin glargine compared with bedtime NPH insulin during insulin combination therapy in type 2 diabetes. *Diabetes Care* **23**: 1130–6.

Yki-Jarvinen H, Kauppinen-Mkelin R, Tiikkainen M, *et al.* (2006) Insulin glargine or NPH combined with metformin in type 2 diabetes: the LANMET study. *Diabetologia* **49**: 442–51.

Yki-Jarvinen H, Juurinen L, Alvarsson M, *et al.* (2007) Initiate Insulin by Aggressive Titration and Education (INITIATE): a randomised study to compare initiation of insulin combination therapy in type 2 diabetic patients individually and in groups. *Diabetes Care* **30**: 1364–9.

Chapter 10

Challenges to good diabetes care

Cathy E Lloyd, Jill Hill, Jackie Webb
and Abd A Tahrani

> **Key points**
> - Good diabetes care requires a partnership approach between the multi-disciplinary professional team and the person with diabetes
> - There are a number of challenges to providing appropriate diabetes care, for both the person with the condition and the health-care professionals involved
> - The National Service Framework for diabetes has provided clear guidelines for the appropriate delivery of care
> - There are specific concerns with regard to the management of diabetes in minority ethnic groups which can be addressed through person-centred culturally appropriate care
> - Diabetes education, tailored to meet the specific needs of the individual whilst at the same time being widely accessible, has been recommended.

The care of diabetes requires a multi-disciplinary approach, with the person with the condition caring for themselves on a day-to-day basis, in partnership with a number of different health care professionals. This is a sound basis for care but is not without its challenges. There may be multiple demands, with a wide range of self-care behaviours expected to be performed, and numerous complications (acute and chronic) that might be experienced, all of which may require the help and support of the health care team.

Working together in partnership along with the wide range of needs of each individual with diabetes implies a holistic approach to care; an approach that recognizes the need for taking the whole person in to account.

Diabetes brings with it an increased risk of a range of both physical and psychological problems, such as depression and anxiety (Lustman *et al.*, 1998; Lloyd, 2000, 2010, 2010a). Having a long-term condition such as diabetes also has implications for employment opportunities, social and personal relationships, as well as the possibility of disability and the often accompanying stigma and social exclusion.

Diabetes, its complications and the side effects of treatment can have a negative impact on quality of life. In the UKPDS, the presence of microvascular complications resulted in worse general health, more mobility problems, more problems with usual activity, more tension, and more mood disturbances (UKPDS Group, 1999). Hypoglycaemic episodes resulted in more tension, more mood disturbance and less work satisfaction. More recent studies have also shown a significant association between depressive symptoms and the presence of diabetes related complications (de Groot *et al.*, 2001; Lloyd *et al.*, 2010). Depression has been found to be associated with the presence of a range of diabetes complications including retinopathy, nephropathy, neuropathy, sexual dysfunction and macrovascular disease (de Groot *et al.*, 2001). In another study the experience of severe hypoglycaemia was associated with increased worry scores (Hoey *et al.*, 2001). Indeed the presence of acute complications has been universally associated with worsening of quality of life (Jacobson, 2004).

Improvement in the care delivered to people with diabetes reduces the development of complications and improves quality of life. This was clearly demonstrated by the findings of the UKPDS, which showed that intensive measures taken to improve glycaemic and blood pressure control resulted in improvements in quality of life.

The National Service Framework (NSF) for diabetes has had important implications for both people with diabetes and the health care professionals involved in their management. A partnership approach to care is advocated, but this implies knowledge and understanding of diabetes and how to achieve optimum standards of care on both sides. A wide range of health care personnel could potentially be involved in this care, including physicians, nurses, health care assistants, dieticians, and podiatrists, working alongside the individual with the condition itself as well as their family. There is the potential for duplication of care, omission of care (if a health care professional assumes someone else is providing that aspect of care) and the delivery of mixed and conflicting advice to the person with diabetes in the centre of this care. See also Box 10.1.

10.1 **Behavioural change**

Prochaska and DiClemente (2003) have developed a model of behaviour change, called the Stages of Change Model, that can be of

> **Box 10.1 National Service Framework (NSF) for diabetes 'Standard 3: Empowering people with diabetes'**
>
> All children, young people and adults with diabetes will receive a service which encourages partnership in decision-making, supports them in managing their diabetes and helps them adopt and maintain a healthy lifestyle. This will be reflected in an agreed and shared care plan in an appropriate format and language. Where appropriate, parents and carers should be fully engaged in this process.
>
> (Department of Health 2001, p. 5).

use in diabetes care. This identifies multiple stages that patients go through, sometimes for many cycles, in order to achieve a change in behaviour (Bundy, 2004) (Figure 10.1). These stages include:

- pre-contemplation, when the individual is not considering change
- contemplation, when they are favourably prepared to change but have not made definite plans
- planning, when strategies have been selected but not yet used
- action, when attempts have been made to change behaviour
- maintenance, when people make deliberate attempts to continue with the change programme.

The model differentiates between a lapse (a temporary return to the previous behaviour) and a relapse (a permanent return to the behaviour being changed).

It is important to identify that people are not always unwilling to change behaviour, but rather they may perceive the suggested behaviour change to be of little benefit to them. If advice is framed from the healthcare professionals' perspective and not the patient's, the patient

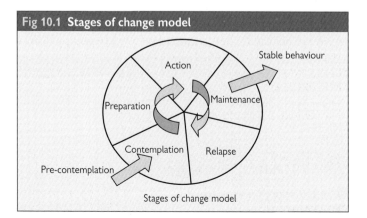

Fig 10.1 Stages of change model

Stable behaviour

Action

Maintenance

Preparation

Contemplation

Relapse

Pre-contemplation

Stages of change model

may perceive the recommendation to be inappropriate for them and therefore be unlikely to take up the advice or change behaviour.

Motivation is a state of readiness to change (Bundy, 2004) and therefore comes at the contemplation stage of the Prochaska and DiClemente model. Motivational interviewing is a person-centred cognitive–behavioral technique that aims to help patients identify and change behaviors that put them at risk or prevent optimal management of a chronic condition.

Miller and Rollnick outlined the steps of motivational interviewing (Bundy, 2004), as detailed in Box 10.2.

Further reading regarding behavioural change and motivational interviewing can be found in multiple publications by Prochaska and DiClemente.

The partnership approach to care implies that health care professionals and the person with diabetes should work together towards commonly agreed goals in order to optimize care and improve outcomes. As laid out in the third of the 12 standards set out in the NSF, empowering people with diabetes is the key to a partnership approach.

The principle of empowerment in diabetes care is based upon people taking more control of their care, both for themselves as individuals, and also for others being involved in determining local services and priorities (Anderson & Funnell, 2000). An empowerment approach to care takes into account social, psychological and environmental factors as well as medical ones. Hiscock (2001) identified a set of factors that contribute to a positive experience in diabetes care, which included a willingness to understand the impact of diabetes on other aspects of the individual's life and lifestyle.

Anderson and Funnell (2000) have compared two models of diabetes care, which are reproduced in Table 10.1. They compared an empowerment model with what they called a 'traditional model' of care, and identified the differences in styles of care in terms of providing diabetes education. Diabetes education, usually provided by nurses, is the cornerstone of diabetes care and includes not only knowledge and information dissemination but skills and confidence

---

Box 10.2 Stages of motivational interviewing

- Establishing rapport
- Setting the agenda
- Assessing readiness to change
- Sharpening the focus
- Identifying ambivalence
- Eliciting self-motivating statements
- Handling resistance
- Shifting the focus.

Table 10.1 Two models of diabetes education

The empowerment model	The traditional model
1 Diabetes is a bio-psychosocial illness.	1 Diabetes is a physical illness.
2 Relationship of provider and patient is democratic and based on shared expertise.	2 Relationship of provider and patient is authoritarian based on provider expertise.
3 Problems and learning needs are usually identified by the patient.	3 Problems and learning needs are usually identified by professional.
4 Patient is viewed as problem solver and caregiver, i.e. professional acts as a resource and helps the patient set goals and develop a self-management plan.	4 Professional is viewed as problem solver and caregiver, i.e., professional responsible for diagnosis and outcome.
5 Goal is to enable patients to make informed choices. Behavioural strategies are used to help patients experiment with behaviour changes of their choosing. Behaviour changes that are not adopted are viewed as learning tools to provide new information that can be used to develop future plans and goals.	5 Goal is behaviour change. Behavioural strategies are used to increase compliance with recommended treatment. A lack of compliance is viewed as a failure of patient and provider.
6 Behaviour changes are internally motivated.	6 Behaviour changes are externally motivated.
7 Patient and professional are powerful.	7 Patient is powerless, professional is powerful.

(Adapted from Anderson & Funnell, 2000, p. 43)

building in order for each individual to feel able to carry out diabetes self-care activities.

The use of an empowerment approach to diabetes care may seem straightforward to some practitioners. However, for others, given the huge variability in patient need, type of diabetes care regimen and external factors that might influence self-care, the implications may seem daunting. It implies that during each consultation between the person with diabetes and a health care professional, a dialogue should take place during which these factors can be taken into account, and suggests that all those involved are able to communicate effectively within the time constraints of a consultation.

A partnership approach to diabetes care is also recommended by government bodies, Diabetes UK, and many others working within the field of diabetes. However, this may appear to be difficult to attain in some circumstances. In particular, these aims and goals may be difficult to achieve when working with particular sections of the diabetes population. Given the increasing prevalence of diabetes in people from minority ethnic backgrounds, working with and understanding the issues and particular concerns of individuals from minority ethnic backgrounds has become of greater concern. For example, the risk of Type 2 diabetes is known to be greater in minority ethnic groups, such as in the South Asian communities in the UK (Barnett et al., 2006; Khunti et al., 2009). There are also a number of particular problems with regard to the management of the condition in this group. In particular, cultural and communication difficulties often make appropriate support of self-management of diabetes more difficult (Greenhalgh, 1998; Lloyd 2006, 2008). However, a small study recently demonstrated that the use of Asian Support Workers, or Asian Link Workers, markedly improves patient outcomes, in terms of increased knowledge and understanding of their diabetes, improved attendance rates at clinics and at education sessions (Curtis et al., 2003). An understanding of cultural difference is important. However, it is vital that difference is not assumed on the basis of appearance or language. Diversity is present within as well as between different cultural groups and an understanding of individual needs and concerns remains key if self-care is to be optimized.

Both physical and psychological complications may occur as a result of having diabetes, and diabetes care is affected by psychological and emotional well-being. In recent years there has been a heightened interest in psychological well-being and diabetes, and research has shown that depressed mood is more common in people with diabetes compared to those without the condition (Lloyd et al., 2010, 2010a, Anderson et al., 2001, Nouwen et al., 2010). Psychological well-being impacts on self-care, for example depressed mood often leads to poor dietary management, lack of physical activity, and poor health behaviours such as increased smoking and alcohol intake. Depressed mood is also associated with an increase in the hormone cortisol which leads to increases in blood glucose levels and thereby poorer glycaemic control. This in turn can lead to an increased risk of developing diabetes complications. Unfortunately, depression is often undiagnosed and therefore untreated, but antidepressant therapy has been shown to be effective and has been found to be associated with improved levels of glycaemic control, often in combination with other therapies such as cognitive behavioural therapy (Lustman et al., 1998, van der Feltz-Cornelis, 2010). The NSF for diabetes recognized the importance of addressing the psychological consequences of illness (DoH, 2001, p. 22), and the National Institute for Health & Clinical Excellence (NICE, 2004) have provided a framework in which to organize the provision of services for treating depression, supporting patients/carers and healthcare professionals in identifying and accessing the most effective interventions. However, as reported by Diabetes UK, in their State of the Nation report (2005), many people felt the provision of emotional support was still a significant gap in diabetes services, particularly for children, young people and parents (Diabetes UK, 2005). This was underscored in a recent report which found that psychological services for people with diabetes remained scarce (Nicholson et al., 2009).

Given the plethora of research demonstrating the importance of psychological well being in those with diabetes, and the official guidance in terms of screening as well as treating psychological problems, this has serious implications for the health care professionals working with those with diabetes. The Diabetes UK State of the Nations report (2005) stated that 'All people with diabetes need access to psychological and emotional support . . . so that they can manage their condition effectively and reduce the risk of complications' (Diabetes UK 2005, p. 31). Furthermore the access to psychological and emotional support should come 'from healthcare professionals with the appropriate skills. . . .' (p. 31). In order to meet those needs however, greater resources need to be invested to increase access to specialist psychological and emotional support for people with diabetes, as well as training in order to carry out screening and referral procedures for those identified as being at risk (NHS Diabetes/Diabetes UK, 2010).

At the time the NSF for diabetes was published, it was increasingly recognized that current approaches to diabetes care, in the UK and around the world, were not realizing the outcomes that would be expected based on the development of new drugs and treatment regimens. Many large scale surveys reported that the majority of people with diabetes do not reach or maintain their goals for diabetes care, even with intensive support, and good metabolic control often remains elusive. For some commentators, the answer to this problem lies within notions of 'non-adherence' or 'non-compliance'. The concept of compliance implies that the patient is a passive recipient of doctors' orders; the doctor being the person with the knowledge of 'what's best' for the patient. Non-compliance therefore is seen to occur when the patient does not follow doctors' orders and, in the case of diabetes, does not perform recommended self-management behaviours such as testing blood sugars, medication taking and dietary self-management. The concept of non-compliance may not necessarily be a helpful one when trying to understand how individuals look after themselves however. Indeed, as Lerner argued, in a review of the literature on non-compliance, 'labels such as 'non-compliant' are invariably judgmental' (Lerner, 1997, p. 1423).

In recent years there has been a further rejection of the notion of non-compliance in favour of 'concordance' (Ferner, 2003). Proponents of concordance argue that this is a far preferable term as it promotes constructive dialogue between patient and health-care professional. This dialogue includes discussion of the risks and benefits of any medication taking or other self-care activities, and forms the basis on which any decisions on the part of patient can be made. It is important to recognize that concordance with recommendations for self-care may be varied; even though insulin may be injected at the appropriate times, or other diabetes medication taken, this does not mean that other vital aspects of diabetes self-care are performed.

People with diabetes may be willing/able to perform different self-care behaviours at different times and structural and/or environmental factors may impact on self-management.

Type 2 diabetes is a complex condition and polypharmacy to address hypertension, dyslipidaemia as well as hyperglycaemia is usually required. If diabetes is seen as a 'sugar disease', individuals may not be aware of the importance of managing blood pressure and lipids as part of their diabetes treatment. Often, the person with type 2 diabetes has few noticeable symptoms and so may not be motivated to take their medication as prescribed as they may feel no different whether they remember to take it or not. Indeed, the medication may have side effects, which results in them feeling less well when they take medication regularly (e.g. gastro-intestinal problems with metformin, hypoglycaemia and weight gain with sulfonylureas and insulin). The Diabetes Audit and Research in Tayside Scotland study (DARTS) demonstrated that a significant number of people with diabetes did not take their medication as prescribed. This worsened as the number of dosing times per day increased (Donnan et al., 2002).

The notions of empowerment, concordance and compliance share some assumptions with regard to how much knowledge of diabetes and diabetes care each individual person with the condition holds. Ideally each person with diabetes should be offered structured diabetes education, either in a group or on an individual basis (NICE, 2003). The National Institute for Health and Clinical Excellence (NICE) have advocated that diabetes education should be tailored to meet the specific needs of individuals, whilst at the same time being 'accessible to the broadest range of people, taking into account culture, ethnicity, disability and geographical issues' (NICE, 2003, p. 4). This is indeed a challenge for the providers of diabetes education, given the variability in terms of not only diabetes knowledge, but all the factors listed above.

For most people with type 2 diabetes, weight management and increasing physical activity are key to addressing the insulin resistance that contributes to hyperglycaemia, hypertension, and dyslipidaemia that characterizes the condition. This usually involves the patient being advised to make a number of lifestyle and behaviour changes at an age when daily behaviours are well established. Eating a healthy diet, increasing physical activity, stopping smoking and reducing alcohol intake may be difficult to achieve and even more difficult to maintain. Difficulties in achieving some of these goals was recognized in people who participated in the DAWN (Diabetes Attitudes Wishes and Needs) study (Peyrot et al., 2005). There may be other barriers that make it difficult for patients to follow lifestyle advice. For example, exercise may be avoided if the patient is overweight and they are too embarrassed to be seen in a swimming costume. People with arthritis may find pain and stiffness a barrier to increasing physical activity levels. Effective sign posting to weight management groups, exercise programmes, local walking groups, etc is useful. Encouraging people to begin with a realistic target, to take small steps and build up, and to give feedback and encouragement are all important.

Type 2 diabetes is a complex condition, in which behaviour change and the adoption of a healthy lifestyle is essential for its successful management. This implies that the person with diabetes needs to be well informed about the underlying process of type 2 diabetes, and why and how lifestyle and medication can address the various aspects of the condition, so he or she can make an informed decision about their management. The use of structured education, a supportive multidisciplinary team, clear agreed targets and appropriate feedback are all essential to achieve this. However, it should be recognized that other factors such as depression and cultural differences may be significant barriers to good self-care.

10.2 **Structured education programmes**

10.2.1 **Diabetes Education and Self-Management for Ongoing and Newly Diagnosed (DESMOND)**

DESMOND is a structured group education programme for adults with Type 2 diabetes; it has a theoretical and philosophical base which supports people in identifying their own health risks and responding to them by setting their own specific behavioural goals. A culturally specific version for particular South Asian communities is now available.

More information about DESMOND can be found at: www. desmond-project.org.uk.

10.2.2 **X-PERT**

X-PERT is a six week structured education programme for people with Type 2 diabetes. It is based on the theories of patient empowerment, patient-centred care and activation. X-PERT programmes usually run for 2 hours a week over the six week period. However the programme is flexible and therefore allows adaptation to the specific client group. It meets key criteria to fulfill NICE guidance.

More information can be found at www.xperthealth.org.uk.

10.2.3 **Other programmes and sources of information**

There are other programmes for people with Type 2 diabetes, details of which can be accessed easily online. One such programme is Me2 from Bolton; this is a system that supports people to live well with diabetes in their everyday life. It provides a platform for people to co-create care services with professionals that are right for them as individuals. The system is based on Agenda cards which reframe the interaction between patients and professionals, giving patients the agenda—this fits well with motivational interviewing.

Other systems are based upon telephone support which enables the patient to develop mastery through reflecting on their successes with an informed and trusted individual who can also offer verbal encouragement. There is also the buddy system, the aim of which is to introduce a process of patient involvement that will, where requested, support and reassure people with diabetes in their understanding and self management of the condition. Buddies are specially trained and receive education in communication, awareness of diabetes, different concepts of care and self management and a code of practice. The national Expert Patient Programme is also available and aims to help people with long term conditions, including diabetes, manage their condition (http://www.nhs.uk/conditions/Expert-patients-programme-/Pages/Introduction.aspx). The basis of the programme is a generic training course that encourages people to manage their condition through developing five core skills:

- problem solving
- decision making
- making the best use of resources
- developing effective partnerships with healthcare providers
- taking appropriate action.

Other resources for both practitioners and people with diabetes include the Diabetes UK website (www.diabetes.org.uk), the Open University short course *Diabetes Care*, details of which can be found at www3.open.ac.uk/study/undergraduate/course/sk120.htm, and www.healthtalkonline.org/, a web-based charity where service user experiences of long-term conditions can be accessed.

10.3 **Summary and conclusions**

Diabetes mellitus is a major challenge to the UK with rising prevalence and significant impact on patients and the NHS. A multidisciplinary approach is vital to fight this epidemic and patient involvement is essential. Health professionals should provide adequate support and education to patients so they can take an active lead in managing their condition. Management plans should be individually tailored in order to meet patient needs taking into account their circumstances, education and culturally specific factors. Behavioural change plays an important role in managing diabetes. Understanding the cycle of change is essential in order to encourage patients to change their behaviour successfully.

References

Anderson RJ, Freedland KE, Clouse RE, Lustman PJ (2001) The prevalence of comorbid depression in adults with diabetes: a meta-analysis. *Diabetes Care* **24**: 1069–78.

Anderson RM, Funnell MM (2001) *The Art of Empowerment*, Alexandria, American Diabetes Association.

Barnett AH, Dixon AN, Bellary S, Hanif MW, O'Hare JP, Raymond NT, Kumar S (2006) Type 2 diabetes and cardiovascular risk in the UK South Asian community. *Diabetologia* **49**: 2234–46.

Bundy C (2004) Changing behaviour: using motivational interviewing techniques. *JR Soc Med* **97**: 43–7.

Curtis S, Beirne J, Jude E (2003) Advantages of training Asian diabetes support workers for Asian families and diabetes health care professionals. *Practical Diabetes International* **20**: 215–18.

De Groot M, Andreson R, Freedland KE, Clouse RE, Lustman PJ (2001) Association of depression and diabetes complications: a meta-analysis. *Psychosom Med* **63**: 619–30.

Department of Health (2001) National Service Framework for Diabetes. London, Department of Health.

Department of Health (2002) NSF for Diabetes Standards of Core Document 2002. www.doh.gov.uk/nsf/diabetes/.

Department of Health (2002) National Service Framework for Diabetes: Delivery strategy. London, Department of Health.

Diabetes UK (2005) State of the Nations 2005: progress made in delivering the national diabetes frameworks. www.diabetes.org.uk/Documents/Reports/StateOfNations.pdf (accessed 1 September, 2010).

Donnan PT, MacDonald TM, Morris AD (2002) Adherence to prescribed oral hypoglycaemic medication in a population of patients with type 2 diabetes: a retrospective cohort study. *Diabetes Medicine* **19**: 278–84.

Ferner, RE (2003) Editorial: Is concordance the primrose path to health? *BMJ* **327**: 821–2.

Greenhalgh T, Helman C, Chowdhury AM (1998) Health beliefs and folk models of diabetes in British Bangladeshis: a qualitative study. *BMJ* **316**: 978–83.

Hiscock J, Legard R, Snape D (2001) Listening to diabetes service users: qualitative findings for the National Service Framework. London, Department of Health.

Hoey H, Aanstood HJ, Chiarelli F, *et al.* (2001) Good metabolic control is associated with better quality of life in 2101 adolescents with Type 1 diabetes. *Diabetes Care* **24**: 1923–8.

Jacobson AM (2004) Impact of improved glycaemic control on quality of life in patients with diabetes. *Endocr Pract* **10**: 502–8.

Khunti K, Kumar S and Brodie (eds) (2009) Diabetes UK and South Asian Health Foundation recommendations on diabetes research priorities for British South Asians. Diabetes UK, London.

Lerner, B (1997) From careless consumptives to recalcitrant patients: the historical construction of non-compliance. *Soc Sci Med* **45**: 1423–31.

Lloyd CE, Dyer PH, Barnett AH (2000) Prevalence of symptoms of depression and anxiety in a diabetes clinic population. *Diabetic Medicine* **17**: 198–202.

Lloyd CE, Mughal S, Sturt J, O'Hare P, Barnett AH (2006) Using self-complete questionnaires in a South Asian population with diabetes: problems and solutions. *Diversity in Health & Social Care* **3**: 245–51.

Lloyd CE, Sturt J, Johnson MRD, Mughal S, Collins G and Barnett AH (2008) Development of alternative modes of data collectionin South Asians with Type 2 diabetes. *Diabetic Medicine* **25**: 455–62.

Lloyd CE, Underwood L, Winkley K, Nouwen A, Hermanns N, Pouwer F (2010) The epidemiology of diabetes and depression. In: Katon W, Sartorius N and Maj M (eds) *Depression and Diabetes*, Wiley/Blackwell.

Lloyd CE (2010a) Diabetes and mental health; the problem of co-morbidity. *Diabetic Medicine Editorial* **12**: 853–4.

Lustman PJ, Griffith LS, Freedland KE, Kissel SS, Clouse RE (1998) Cogntive behaviour therapy for depression in type 2 diabetes mellitus. A randomized controlled trial. *Ann Int Med* **129**: 61–621.

NHS Diabetes and Diabetes UK (2010) Emotional and psychological support and care in diabetes. Report from the emotional and psychologycal support working group of NHS Diabetes and Diabetes UK.

NICE (2003) Guidance on the use of patient-education models for diabetes. Technology appraisal 60. National Institute for Health and Clinical Excellence, London.

NICE (2004) Management of depression in primary and secondary care. Clinical guideline 23, National Institute for Health and Clinical Excellence, London.

Nicholson TRJ, Taylor J-P, Gosden C, Trigwell P, Ismail K (2009) National guidelines for psychological care in diabetes: how mindful have we been? *Diabetic Med* **26**: 447–50.

Nouwen A, Winkley K, Twisk J, Lloyd CE, Peyrot M, Ismail K, Pouwer F (2010) Type 2 Diabetes Mellitus as a risk factor for the onset of depression: a systematic review and meta-analysis. *Diabetologia* (In Press).

Peyrot M, Rubin RR, Lauritzen T (2005) Psychological problems and barriers to improved diabetes management: results of the Cross-National Diabetes Attitudes, Wishes and Needs (DAWN) study. *Diabetes Medicine* **22**: 1379–85.

UK Prospective Diabetes Study Group (1999) Quality of life in type 2 diabetic patients is affected by complications but not by intensive policies to improve blood glucose or blood pressure control. *Diabetes Care* **22**: 1125–36.

van der Feltz-Cornelis, C, Nuyen J, *et al* (2010) Effect of interventions for major depressive disorder and significant depressive symptoms in patients with diabetes mellitus: a systematic review and meta-analysis. *Gen Hosp Psychiatry* **32**: 380–95.

Index

Note: page numbers in *italics* refer to Figures and Tables.